THE
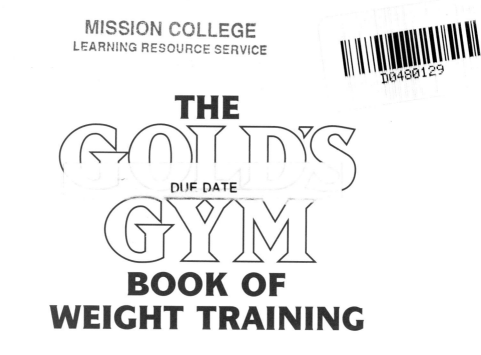
GOLD'S
DUE DATE
GYM
BOOK OF
WEIGHT TRAINING

Other books by Ken Sprague

SPORTS STRENGTH
THE ATHLETE'S BODY
THE GOLD'S GYM BOOK OF BODYBUILDING
THE GOLD'S GYM BOOK OF STRENGTH TRAINING
WEIGHT AND STRENGTH TRAINING FOR KIDS AND TEENAGERS

THE GOLD'S GYM

BOOK OF
WEIGHT TRAINING

Ken Sprague

Photography by John Bauguess

A Perigee Book

To Maryon, Pete, Ed, and Tim—
who built a golden oak from a single acorn

Perigee Books
are published by
The Putnam Publishing Group
200 Madison Avenue
New York, NY 10016

Library of Congress Cataloging-in-Publication Data
Sprague, Ken.
   The Gold's Gym Book of weight training / Ken Sprague ; photography by
John Bauguess.
      p. cm.
   "A Perigee book."
   ISBN 0-399-51846-0
   1. Weight training. I. Title.
GV546.S68 1994
613.7'13—dc20   93-5839 CIP

Cover design by Andrew M. Newman
Front cover photograph copyright © 1993 by John Bauguess

Printed in the United States of America
         4 5 6 7 8 9 10

This book is printed on acid-free paper.
                  ∞

The weight training routines in this book are intended for healthy individuals. People with health problems should not follow these routines without a physician's approval. Before beginning any exercise or nutrition program, always consult with your doctor. Children should always be supervised by an adult while performing these exercises.

CONTENTS

ACKNOWLEDGMENTS

The original edition of *The Gold's Gym Book of Weight Training* was the idea of Jeremy Tarcher, without whose help the Gold's Gym weight training program would never have found a literary format. Many evenings were spent in the middle of the Tarcher living room, developing text and corresponding photographs. He deserves top billing among all who have contributed to this project.

Thanks too to Bill Dobbins for his contributions of doggedly transcribing the ideas of those meetings into prose for the first edition.

There are many contributors to this most recent edition of the *Gold's Gym Book of Weight Training.* The primary photographer, John Bauguess, heads that list: Without photographs, there would be no book.

The photographer's task is made easier by good models. In this case, the models were exceptionally good. Thanks to Bruce Budzig, Patty Chang, Kim Collins, Luis Chicas Cruz, Julie Erdal, Karen Erickson, Amy Fields, Lisa Gladstone, Cynthia Ingstad, Aubree Knecht, Kent Kuehn, Bobby Lamar, Lisa Lyon, Jeff Monroe, Todd Offenbacher, Matt Powers, Jason Randal, Kris Randal, Dusty Sprague, Homer Sprague, Greg Thompson, Kate Weck, Aaron Whitten, Filip Trojanek, Casey Viator, Darlene Wockensky, and Trish Weems for making this a better-looking book.

When a pile of photographs and pages of rough manuscript land on an editor's desk, it takes someone special to piece it together into a cohesive manuscript. I was fortunate to have Laura Shepherd do that for me. Thanks. And a special thanks to Rena Wolner for suggesting a revised edition of this book.

Thanks, Jeremy, Bill, John, Laura, Rena, and all you models for your past and present contributions.

PREFACE

You've picked up this book because you want to look, feel, and perform your very best. This all-new edition—entirely rewritten and illustrated for the 1990s and beyond—will help you do just that.

The Gold's Gym Book of Weight Training provides an easy-to-follow and realistic weight-training program that has already served a generation of women and men worldwide.

The weights are the same. The exercises are the same. But there is one major difference between this edition and that published fifteen years ago. The advice offered in the first edition, derived mostly from my practical experience, has been subsequently supported by a plethora of scientific research.

The Gold's Gym Book of Weight Training is based on my thirty-five years of weight-training experience, and a formal education that includes a Phi Beta Kappa key in science. Along the way, I've coached many champion athletes and bodybuilders with the same training principles that are the foundation of this book. These very principles will allow you to reach your personal training goals.

Part One begins with a brief history of weight training before explaining how weight training interacts with nature, cross-training regimens, and nutrition to build a stronger, fitter, more attractive body. Basic terms, training principles, setting up a home gym, and safety guidelines are also clearly and concisely presented to prepare you for your training program.

Part Two is devoted to training, beginning with a practical Basic Workout of eight exercises incorporating all major muscle groups. Once you've mastered the Basic Workout, spot-training exercises can be added to your workout program. Your personal training goals determine which exercises to add. At the end of Part Two is a chapter devoted to improved sports performance through weight training.

If you're ready to join the legion of successful weight trainers who have taken charge of their bodies, *The Gold's Gym Book of Weight Training* is for you. Use it, rely on it, and share it with others. Feel proud and confident that you're on your way to reaching your fitness goals.

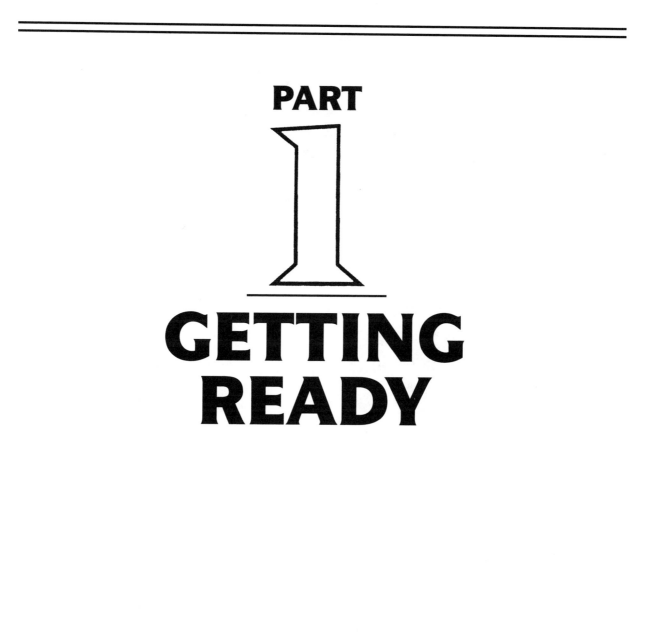

PART

1

GETTING READY

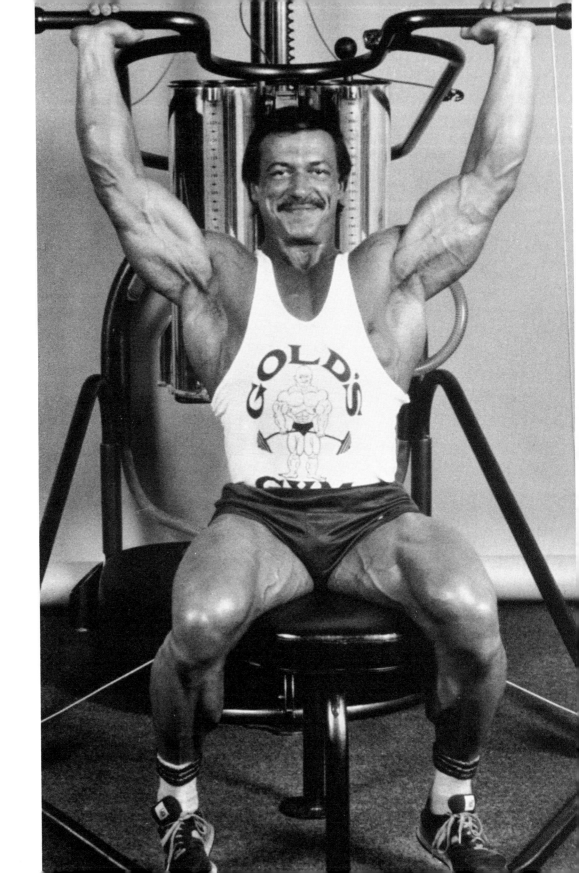

1
A BIT OF HISTORY

The Gold's Gym name is world famous, and has become synonymous with state-of-the-art weight training. That's an amazing accomplishment, considering that the gym has been in existence only since the late 1960s.

The guys of Gold's, an all-male membership at first, didn't invent weight training. That honor is traditionally bestowed on Milo of Crotona, an Olympic-champion wrestler of sixth-century-B.C. Ionia. Each day—so the tale goes—the legendary Milo lifted his pet baby bull. As the bull grew, gained weight, and presumably got meaner, Milo kept lifting him daily and getting stronger.

Milo's 2,500-year-old system of lifting an increasingly heavier bull, known today as progressive resistance training (PRT), is still recognized as the best means to gain strength and sculpt the body. The only substantial difference between Milo's PRT and modern adaptations is the equipment. Barbells and machines, thankfully, have replaced Milo's bull as the equipment of choice.

Milo wasn't the first person to grow stronger from lifting, pushing, or tossing heavy things. Increased strength was a natural consequence of ancient lifestyle. But Milo differed from the hoi polloi of his contemporary society in that he was into recreational strength building. Billions of people who came and went before him didn't much consider the cause-effect relationship between hoisting ever-heavier objects and increased strength. Legends of great strength and heroic feats are found throughout the history of Western cultures. The Hebrews had Sampson and the Ancient Greeks had Ulysses as important symbols of mythology. The exploits of these legendary heroes reflect the importance of a man's physical strength in ancient times.

Amazons aside, physical strength and a muscular form were not revered in women of antiquity. Sampson had Delilah and Ulysses had Penelope, physically weak counterbalances to male virility.

The ideal of the strong muscular male and the soft, weak female persisted into the Renaissance. Michelangelo's David and the male figures adorning the rotunda of the Sistine Chapel are indicative of that period's reverence of the muscular male body. The contemporaneous female ideal was captured by the works of Botticelli and Raphael: soft, delicate forms without a hint of muscularity or strength.

Time marched on. The Victorian era brought a marked change in gender-referenced stereotypes. To be sure, the portrayal of women as weak, delicate creatures continued, and even carried over to portrayals of the male body. Clothing covered almost every inch of skin, and muscles and physical strength were no longer dominant factors in defining the ideal male.

The Victorian change reflected a societal shift from dependence on brute force to a dependence on industrial technology. A muscular physique was evidence of belonging to the working class—a *less powerful* group in a hierarchy increasingly dominated by technological and management skills. Muscles and rough hands were best concealed.

By the 1960s, men who spent countless hours intentionally building muscles—men who worshiped big muscles—were out of sync with history's timeline. They were social outcasts. They were the guys of Gold's. No women or children, they were the *guys* of Gold's.

Later, the women would come in droves, but that's getting ahead of the story.

GOLD'S GYM: A RITE OF PASSAGE

I first heard of Gold's Gym in 1969, shortly after arriving in Venice, California, from Cincinnati. A bodybuilding beach buddy told me about this cheap no-frills gym only a city block from the sands of Venice Beach.

Gold's was indeed a cheap no-frills gym, a storefront with bare concrete floors, block walls, and a collection of homemade and second-hand weight-training equipment. The membership fee—sixty dollars a year—at first seemed high for an overblown garage. But it was close to the sandy, sunny beach. And I, like all bodybuilders, loved the sandy, sunny beach. Muscles and a suntan were complementary vanities.

My first workout at Gold's was spectacular. What the gym lacked in niceties was more than made up for in atmosphere. In fact, the atmosphere was priceless. There was no other place on earth that could match it for a bodybuilder.

The atmosphere evolved from the hundred-or-so pioneering members of Gold's Gym united by hard-core bodybuilding—a maelstrom of madness that valued a rippled, muscular appearance above all else; a madness elevated to an art form by an intense, competitive training environment. Who had the biggest arms, the best abs, the best chest? Gold's fostered an obsessive, competitive, self-absorbed madness. An obsession with mirrors. An obsession with self.

Outside the gym, the Southern California sun and 1960s bohemian lifestyle of Venice Beach were hospitable to bodybuilders. Make no mistake, during the 1960s bodybuilders were social outcasts in Boston, Portland, and Cincinnati. But outcasts of all types were welcome in Venice. Hell's Angels, drug dealers, religious fanatics, artists, and bodybuilders got along as one huge, diverse community of misfits. From that perspective, the hulking bodybuilders were Venice mainstream. Gold's was in the middle of it all.

On the inside, Gold's Gym was a clubhouse, a safe haven for kindred spirits, a place of physical spirituality. Most of the early members had been bodybuilding champions in their hometowns. Titles abound: Mr. Massachusetts, Mr. Oregon, and so on—and even me, Mr. Cincinnati.

Atop the gym's pecking order were the Mr. America and Mr. Universe winners, the kings of muscledom. But they were celebrated only in the gym. One in-house celebrity, unknown even in east Venice, was a young Arnold Schwarzenegger, who had only recently immigrated from Austria. International celebrity would be his future, but in 1969, only a handful of hard-core bodybuilders had heard of Arnold—or Gold's for that matter.

The popularity of Gold's Gym and Arnold was slow to develop. A case in point is the first Gold's-sponsored bodybuilding show. The year was 1972. Fewer than fifty spectators, including family and friends of contestants, would pay five dollars for a ticket. Arnold, the headline act (guest poser), was paid $50 for his efforts. What later became marquee names—Gold's Gym and Arnold Schwarzenegger—couldn't draw enough spectators to recoup the five-hundred-dollar investment of that first show. That was the plight of bodybuilding and bodybuilders in the early 1970s.

By 1977, fortunes were changing. Arnold was on the path of an

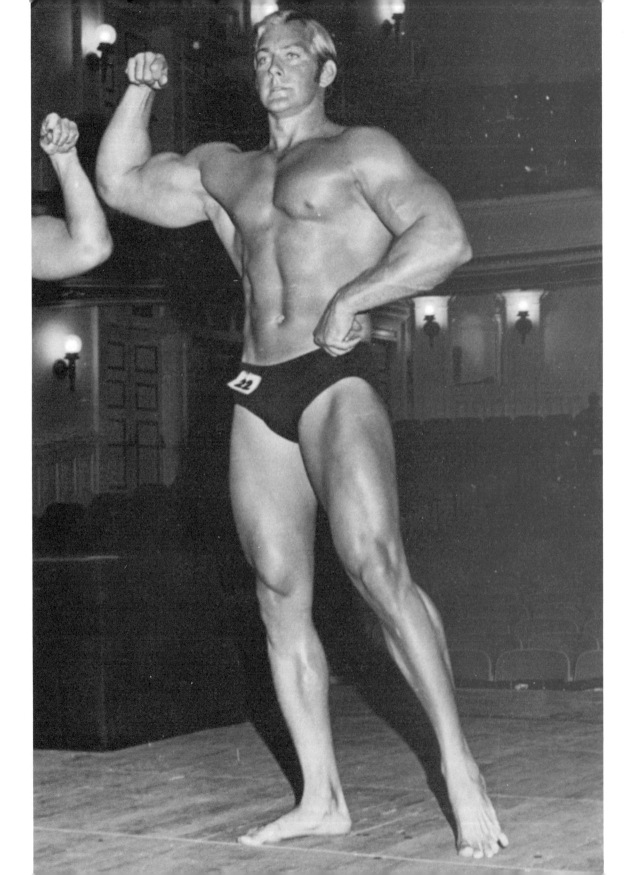

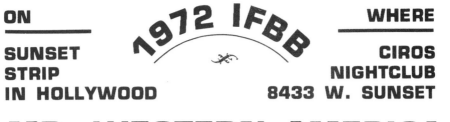
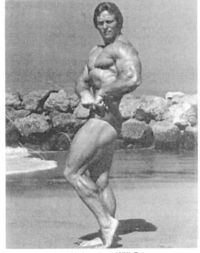
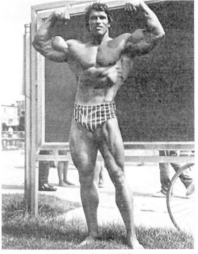
1972 Contest Poster

Ken Sprague, 1967 Mr. Cincinnati

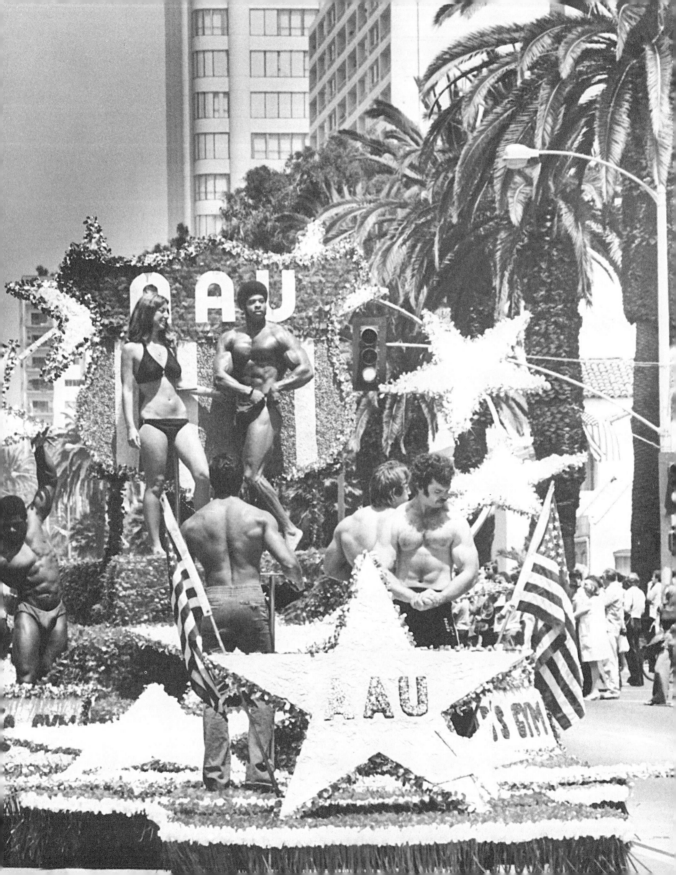

acting career, gaining mainstream attention through the promotion of *Pumping Iron,* a documentary film on bodybuilding. Gold's, the primary location for that film, shared the limelight.

Gold's Gym was gaining attention through other vehicles, too. The 1977 Mr. America contest, a Gold's production, drew a quarter-million spectators for the "Bodybuilding Day Parade." Six thousand paying spectators cheered as Mae West crowned the new Mr. America that evening. Media coverage rivaled that of the Academy Awards show that year. Hundreds of media outlets, as diverse as *60 Minutes* and *National Geographic,* splashed images of Gold's Gym and its menagerie of bodybuilders to millions of viewers worldwide. Gold's Gym had become the undisputed mecca of bodybuilding.

More contests and extensive media coverage would follow. And that onslaught of publicity precipitated an expanded public interest in weight training as a legitimate fitness activity. The end result: That small collection of bodybuilders training in a concrete bunker only a quarter-century ago has been joined by 35 million weight trainers throughout the United States, and millions more worldwide. Arnold, once an unknown Austrian bodybuilder with gapped teeth and unworkable accent, is now an international superstar. Gold's Gym now boasts four hundred locations that dot the globe.

In a quarter of a century, weight training has grown from a minor footnote to a mainstay on the American fitness scene. Gold's led the way among gyms, for women as well as men.

WOMEN JOIN WEIGHT TRAINING

In retrospect it seems trite, but one of my toughest early decisions as owner of Gold's Gym involved a woman. The year was 1972. A woman wanted to join.

Nearly unanimous among the all-male membership was the opinion that allowing "girls" to train on the hallowed grounds of Gold's was a sacrilege. Girls and weight training? Ugh!

Cutting the story short, that determined young woman became the first female to train at Gold's Gym. She was one of a relatively few women weight trainers anywhere in the country at that time.

Other adventurous women would soon join the gym. One of those was Lisa Lyon, winner of the first Women's World Bodybuilding Championship in 1979.

Mr. America Parade

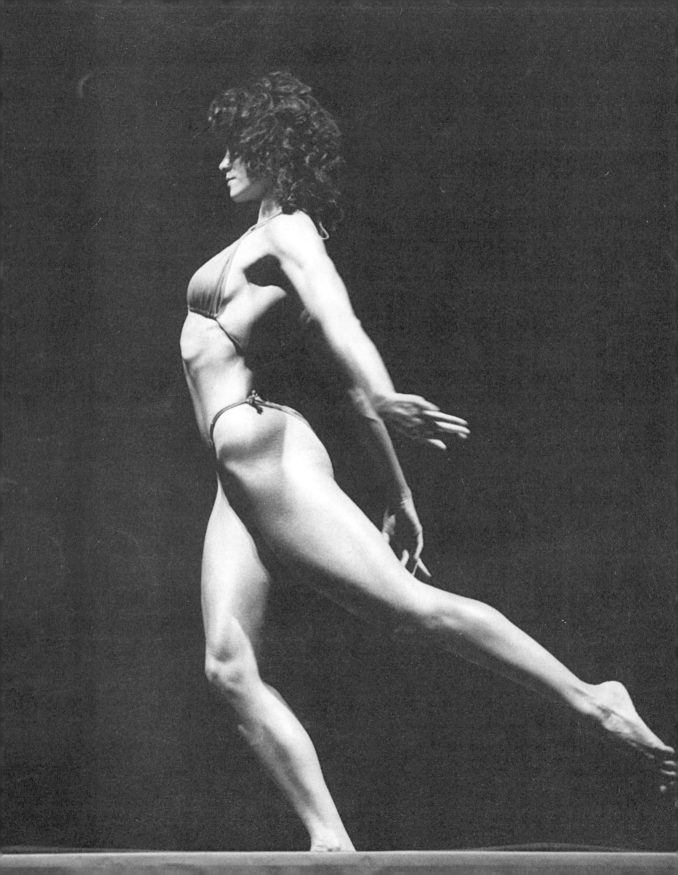

Reflecting a sea of change in female perspective, both mainstream society and the weight-training world has turned on its axis in the last twenty-five years for women, who often outnumber men in the weight room today. Women's weight training has hit full stride. And why not? The benefits of weight training are nondiscriminatory.

TODAY'S ATHLETIC LOOK

In a nutshell, Arnold's dramatic increase in earning power—from $50 to 15 million dollars as a headline act—reflects the general public's shift in taste: Twenty-five years ago muscles were "out." In the 1990s, a muscular, athletic-looking body is a valued possession.

The nineties woman stands side by side with her athletic male counterpart. Jane Fonda led the revolution in the 1980s. Cindy Crawford, Linda Hamilton, and Demi Moore pump iron in the 1990s. A new definition of femininity has emerged along the way as the stars act as beacons for the rest of us. The "soft," "voluptuous" look of the past has been replaced by today's lean, athletic look.

THE GROWTH IN POPULARITY OF WEIGHT TRAINING

Why the exponential growth in weight training? That's easy to answer: Because it works. Here's how:

Sculpting the Body
Weight training is the only fitness activity that can selectively reproportion the body. Want more shapely calves? There are exercises specifically designed to change the shape and size of the calf. How about wider shoulders? There are exercises designed specifically to add width to the shoulders. In fact, there are specific exercises for every body part. You become both an artist and a living piece of sculpture, adding a little here and removing a little there. Unlike Michelangelo, you can carry the fruits of your labor with you twenty-four hours a day.

Self-esteem
There's no getting around the fact that vanity is endemic to our collective American personality—why else would you care so much about

Lisa Lyon, first Women's World Champion

how you look? Yes, you could rationalize paying attention to your appearance as a social necessity. But whichever perspective you choose, *your* perception of how you look is a major component of *your* self-esteem. Face it, feeling fat and out of shape is a downer; feeling trim and fit feels great!

Body image often affects the rest of our personality. Knowing that you "look good" boosts positive self-esteem. Positive self-esteem established through an improved body image carries over into multiple activities.

Improved self-esteem can be a major benefit of weight training. The positive physical change induces positive psychological change. You look better and you know it. You're brimming with confidence.

Strength

Increased strength is the most obvious benefit of weight training. Not as obvious is the enormous breadth of applications of that increased strength.

A stronger athlete is a better athlete. A stronger shoulder girdle improves the posture, elevating the breasts. Stronger arms and legs make an easier task of carrying out the garbage. Strength builds confidence. Strength provides access to a wider range of jobs. Strength prevents injury. Strength enhances numerous activities, opens a multitude of opportunities, and eases some of life's obstacles.

THE PRESENT AND FUTURE OF WEIGHT TRAINING

Today, you're likely to find yourself weight training side by side with a doctor, lawyer, teacher, secretary, student, or sports star. The diversity of today's gym membership stands in stark contrast to yesterday's all-male bastions of hard-core bodybuilding. But the goals of all members are similar. They all seek the wide range of benefits that weight training can provide.

How will the future of weight training unfold? With millions of men and women now weight training for a stronger, leaner, more fit body, the next great surge in weight training's popularity is likely to be among children and adolescents. Each day, more and more young people are weight training for sports performance, health, or appearance. High-school and middle-school boys and girls, particularly those concerned with body image and sports performance, are rushing into weight rooms when they learn they can selectively sculpt and strengthen different body parts through this safe, effective activity.

Weight training the Gold's Gym way has worked for millions of people of all ages and both sexes. It worked for Jose Canseco, Michael Jordan, Martina Navratilova, and millions of weekend warriors by making them quicker, stronger, more powerful athletes. It worked for Jane Fonda, Arnold Schwarzenegger, Madonna, Cindy Crawford, as well as millions of ordinary men, women, and children, by sculpting their bodies as only weight training can.

Weight training worked for millions of people by making them feel better about themselves. It can do the same for you.

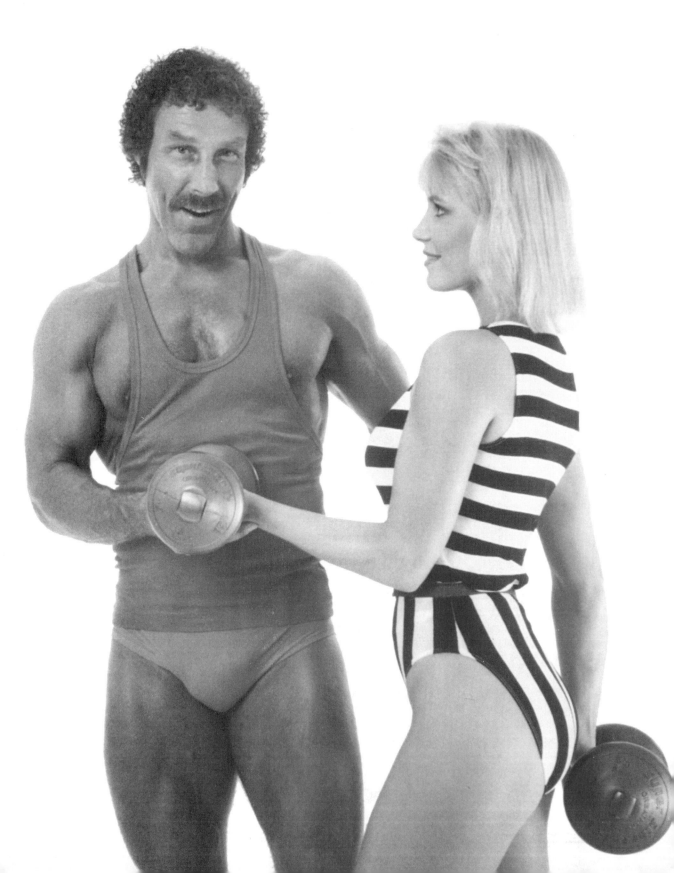

2
WEIGHT TRAINING: HOW IT WORKS

The human body is an all-purpose biological factory bound by cause-effect relationships. Given food, the body converts it to energy. Too much food, it stores the excess energy as fat. Too little food, it draws on stored energy reserves. Too hot, it cools itself. Too cool, it heats itself. Hurt, it repairs itself. In short, it receives information and inventory, and responds with appropriate directives. Let's explore how.

MUSCLES MOVING BONES—THAT'S WEIGHT TRAINING

Mr. Universe reaches down, picks a barbell from the floor, and thrusts it above his head. No problem, right? Wrong. Mr. Universe used several hundred of his more than 600 different muscles to hoist that barbell above his head. Hundreds of muscles synchronously and sequentially pulled on the skeleton to complete the lift. Aptly enough, the muscles involved in that and all other weight-training movements are called *skeletal muscles,* muscles that pull on bones.

Each skeletal muscle is attached to a pair of bones. For example, the biceps muscle is attached to the bones of the upper and lower arm. Bending the arm at the elbow is the responsibility of the biceps muscles. When the brain sends a signal to the biceps to bend the elbow, the biceps shortens, pulling on each of the attached bones, drawing those bones closer together. The result is a bent elbow.

Bending the elbow is simple enough to comphrehend, but imagine the thousands of muscular, bone, and neural interactions that must take place in a fraction of a second to perform a successful lift from floor to overhead. Each message from the brain to each active muscle must be continually revised as bone angles and forces change. But fear not. In a few short months of weight training, your skeletal muscles will perform the most complicated exercises as if they were a well-rehearsed ballet.

WHAT MAKES A MUSCLE GROW?

When Arnold Schwarzenegger was competing as a 240-pound bodybuilder in the 1970s, he had a fifty-eight-inch chest and a twenty-two-inch biceps. Like the rest of us, he started life as a smaller package. How did that baby get *so* big?

Arnold weight trained. In doing so, he added resistance—in the form of barbells and dumbbells—to normal body movements. They were simple movements like raising his hand above his head, bending his knees, and curling his hand toward his shoulder. The same movements he had done with rattles as a baby, but the rattles were later replaced by a barbell and dumbbells. That's weight training in a nutshell—adding resistance to movements that you've been doing all your life.

Arnold's muscles grew and became stronger as an adaptation to the stress of weight training. When a muscle encounters greater resistance than it is accustomed to, a chemical reaction occurs within the muscle that builds more material responsible for that muscle's contractile strength. The result is bigger and stronger muscles.

Through the years, Arnold placed continually greater stress on his muscles by lifting heavier and heavier barbells. As his muscles grew accustomed to a given weight, he added more weight to the barbell. Each additional pound on the barbell caused stronger muscle contractions and correspondingly greater muscle growth. And that little baby grew and grew into a very big boy.

A FEMALE ARNOLD?

No woman will grow Schwarzeneggeresque muscles. She could follow Arnold around the gym duplicating every squat and arm curl, yet never approach his gargantuan proportions. That's because no woman has the same body chemistry as Arnold, particularly his natural supply of a male hormone, testosterone.

The size of an *average* woman's muscles will increase from intensive training, but only to the point of looking athletically fit. Why the emphasis on *average* woman? Because a *few* females do grow big muscles from intense weight training. Female bodybuilding competitions have produced a few striking examples.

There are two primary reasons for these few atypical women. Some are genetic phenomena, having a natural muscle-growing physiology and testosterone levels akin to that of an average male. Others are synthetic phenomena, creating a pseudomale physiology through the use of steroids, which are testosterone derivatives that are injected or ingested to trick the body into growing male-like muscle.

Most women—99.97 percent of them—will not grow massive muscles from intense weight training. A woman's muscles will grow a much smaller amount, contributing to a firm, selectively shaped, stronger, healthier body. That list of benefits, as well as disproving the myth that weight-trained women will grow super-sized muscles, has made weight training a popular fitness activity among women.

BODY SCULPTING: SELECTIVE MUSCLE GROWTH

Weight training can give us a different look. That's because weight training can selectively reshape, or sculpt, your muscles. In fact, weight training is the *only* popular fitness activity that permits you to selectively change your appearance.

Is your goal to add a little to your calves and shoulders? No problem. Weight-training your shoulders and calves will cause that to happen. Want to improve your posture and reshape your thighs and hips? There are weight-training exercises that achieve that too. Weight training, by exploiting your body's cause-effect reaction to training stress, allows you to choose the shape of your body.

Diets won't selectively reshape your body; spot-reducing absolutely won't work. A diet removes fat uniformly from all parts of the body. You get smaller all over. You might lose your saddlebags, but you'll lose your shoulders and breasts, too.

The recommended combination of weight training and diet provides dramatic results. For example, as the diet removes fat from your stomach area, selective weight-training exercises build or retain muscle in your shoulders. The result is a dramatic V-shaped appearance. A redesigned you!

Tired of the way you look? Try a change of muscle.

MUSCLES SHRINK IF UNDERWORKED

Pete Grymkowski, one of the best bodybuilders I have known, reduced his body weight from a muscular 250 pounds to less than 200 pounds. Where did all that muscle go?

It shrank. He quit weight training for a while, and it shrank. Muscles will shrink if not subjected to the high levels of stress to which they've become accustomed. That's because the body won't support unnecessary muscle tissue. The tissue is temporarily phased out, to be rebuilt only if the stresses are again increased by resuming a weight-training program.

How long does it take to *rebuild* the muscle lost during a layoff? Not nearly as long as it takes to build the muscle the first time around. I remember Arnold Schwarzenegger once reducing to about 200 pounds for a role in a movie, *Stay Hungry.* Six weeks later, he had returned to a muscular 235.

MUSCLES CAN GET SORE

Weight training can bring about two types of muscle soreness. The first, *acute* muscle soreness, can occur during weight training if you (mistakenly) engage in sets of super-high reps and intensity. In short, the muscle has insufficient endurance to meet the high-rep training demands. Overextending a muscle's endurance capacity produces an intensely painful burning sensation from lactic-acid buildup. That's what happens to a sprinter's legs during an all-out 400-meter race. Fortunately, the pain quickly subsides as our overworked, energy-depleted muscles recover.

Acute muscle soreness is antithetical to the principles of muscle building and shaping presented in this book. That's because the super-high-rep sets that produce acute soreness don't build or shape muscle.

The second type, *delayed-onset* muscle soreness, earns its name because it strikes from twelve to forty-eight hours following the training session. It's the soreness I experienced after my first aerobics class.

Delayed-onset muscle soreness is common among weight trainers. It is apt to follow a particularly intense or novel workout—novel meaning exercises you perform for the first time.

Delayed-onset muscle soreness is a manifestation of minor injury: If we could peel back the skin covering a sore arm and leg, we would find microscopic tears in the tissue of our muscles, ligaments, and tendons.

Except in extreme cases, soreness is nothing to worry about. The pain will subside in a day or two as the body quickly heals itself.

The best advice to avoid delayed-onset muscle soreness?

1. Follow the principles of progressive resistance training: Gradually increase training demands; slowly increase training resistance over time, progressively overloading the muscle through a sequence of workouts; don't be in a hurry to lift maximum weights, particularly if you're a beginner.

2. When including new exercises in your training routine, start with small weights even if you're capable of lifting far more. Analogous to the previous recommendation, progressively overload the muscles through a sequence of training sessions rather than chancing soreness or a more serious injury that will interrupt your training schedule.

3. Make sure to include a general and first-set warm-up as part of your weight-training program to prepare your muscles for overload training.

4. Follow the recommended exercise technique, particularly in regard to the recommendation of a *controlled* movement. Don't jerk or bounce a barbell or dumbbell. The jerk or bounce increases the effective force on the muscles and joints.

Once soreness occurs, how do you get rid of it? The best advice is to duplicate the exercise that produced the soreness—but with very low intensity. In other words, use very light weights during your next workout.

The increased circulation produced by exercising the sore muscles with light weights will speed recovery by the body's own healing properties.

YOU CAN'T GROW NEW MUSCLES

Mr. America really has no *more* muscles than the latest *Cosmopolitan* model. We're all born with the same number of muscles. And regardless of how hard we train, we can't grow a single new one.

It only looks like people have different muscles. That's because the size of our muscles can differ drastically. For example, it's not uncommon for a male bodybuilder or football lineman to add a hundred pounds of *extra* muscle mass through weight training. But with all that added mass, not one new muscle is created. The same old muscles just increase in size. Like blowing up a package of balloons, the inflated balloons take up more space.

We all have the same number of muscles as the tiniest of babies. How we train them and our sex determines how big and strong they will become.

HIGH DEFINITION: TRAINING AND DIET

A defined, "cut" look demands a combination of weight training and diet. Weight training tones the muscle, while diet removes fat beneath the skin, allowing the toned muscle to stand out. Extreme examples of the diet-exercise regimen are competitive bodybuilders.

On contest night, male and female bodybuilders labor under the spotlight, steel slabs and cables bulging and rippling under cellophane skin. Two days later, those same weight-trained bodies—as much as thirty pounds heavier—have lost that defined, chiseled look. They still have muscle—and something extra, too.

Prior to a contest, most competitive bodybuilders embark on a rigid, months-long diet with the intent of eliminating as much body fat and water as possible. Without the fat and water, particularly subcutaneous fat and water, the muscles show more clearly through the skin. That's definition.

With the contest over, the rigid diet stops. The bodybuilder eats likes the rest of us. The cells manifest a rebound effect, unsure if the hard times of diet will soon be repeated. His or her 30 billion fat cells and water depositories rapidly refill. That's the something extra that can add up to thirty pounds over a two-day period, the something extra that hides those quivering muscles.

The point to be made is that weight training alone, even taken to the extreme of competitive bodybuilding, will not create a super-defined body. A combination of diet and weight training is necessary to do the job. As you will read in the chapter on nutrition, the diet is more reasonable than that followed by a competitive bodybuilder. And if *you* fall off the wagon for a few days, you won't have a rebound effect of a thirty-pound weight gain.

Train hard, diet moderately, and you will have a pleasingly defined body that proudly displays the fruits of your efforts.

WEIGHT TRAINING BUILDS STRONGER BONES

Weight training increases the stress on bones, and bones respond to the added stress as muscles do: by getting bigger and stronger.

How does weight training increase the stress on bones? As the muscles attached to bones are increasingly stressed with heavier and heavier weights, the pull of those muscles on the bones correspondingly increases. The bone responds by growing thicker and denser, adding calcium and phosphorus—the primary bone-building materials.

The bones that receive the most stress add the most strength and thickness. Since a weight trainer can handle the greatest amounts of weights with the muscles of the hips and thighs, these bones will increase the most in thickness and strength.

Does that mean that weight training will give you noticeably thicker hips, thighs, ankles, and knees? No. The changes are imperceptible to the naked eye. Will the bones grow longer, making me taller? No. Weight training won't increase your height, but it can improve your posture, which, in turn, provides a taller "look."

Strengthened bones are a health and fitness advantage. They're less likely to sustain an injury in the case of a trauma from athletic activity or an unexpected slip on the stairs. And exercising to maintain strong bones appears to be particularly important for women, many of whom lose bone integrity through the natural aging process.

There are numerous advantages to training your bones.

THE MOST IMPORTANT RESULT: LIFTING WEIGHTS LIFTS SPIRITS

Perhaps the most dramatic change you will experience through weight training is how you feel about yourself. Improved strength and appearance through weight training translates to improved self-image.

Self-image, or self-esteem, is nurtured through accomplishment. Inevitably, the weight trainer can lift heavier and heavier weights. Lifting heavier weights might at first appear to be unconnected to self-esteem. But lifting the heavier weights offers positive feedback—accomplishment.

A cyclical pattern emerges: As the weight trainer increases strength or muscle tone, his or her self-esteem rises. In short, the improved body image enhances total self-image. Confidence increases in a variety of daily activities. The self-esteem developed with a set of barbells translates into improved self-esteem at school, work, or in a relationship.

Lifting weights lifts spirits.

Body Image and the Adolescent Female

The primary cause of depression among adolescent females is a negative body image.

Few adolescent girls can meet the distorted cultural images of what is "desirable" that are splashed across television and magazines. They can't ignore the distorted message, and are often swept into a cauldron of subliminal comparisons. Body image suffers, self-esteem drops.

Weight training can reverse that cycle.

THE OBVIOUS RESULT OF WEIGHT TRAINING: INCREASED STRENGTH

So close is the connection between strength training and weight training that the terms are often used interchangeably. Undoubtedly, increased strength is a benefit of weight training. But what *happens* within the body that translates to increased strength? That is the question.

The answer depends on the age, sex, and experience of the individual weight trainer.

Traditionally, it was thought that greater strength meant bigger muscles. But studies of beginning weight trainers conducted over the past dozen years have demonstrated amazing strength gains—as much as 100 percent in the first six months of training—without any significant increases in the size of the exercised muscles. How could this happen?

Most exercise theorists believe that *neural adaptations* are the mechanism behind the strength gains of beginning weight trainers. These neural adaptations are improvements in signaling between the brain and the muscle tissue. In short, practicing a weight-training exercise "teaches" more existing muscle tissue to take part in a given movement as stress increases: The muscle always had the capacity to develop the necessary force, but months of training improved the communication from brain to muscle.

Of course, those rapid strength gains don't last forever. The potential for neural adaptations is reached within the first year or so of training. Thereafter, the traditionally recognized mechanism of strength gains (muscle growth) takes over. That's the point at which sex and age are major factors in strength gains.

Strength gains go hand in hand with muscle growth after the exhaustion of neural adaptations. But muscle growth requires testosterone—a hormone in short supply in women and children. Hence, women and children experience *very* slow size and corresponding strength increases even under the most intense training schedules.

A sufficient supply of testosterone allows adult males to continue to gain strength by adding muscle mass after neural adaptations have run their course.

Increased Strength Can Change Your Appearance

Toning and strengthening your muscles, without muscle growth, has a direct effect on how you look. Consider the "stooped shoulder" look, a definite detractor from an attractive posture.

Strengthening the muscles of the shoulder girdle and upper back is corrective action for stooped shoulders, and lifts the breasts as well.

It's as simple as one, two, three. Three exercises—upright rows, dumbbell presses, and shrugs—strengthen the muscles that cause the physical lift, while uplifting your spirits as well.

OVERVIEW: A STRONGER BODY AND MIND

Weight training can improve your strength, appearance, and self-esteem through a cause-effect relationship. Specific exercises cause specific muscles to change shape and strengthen. Implementing a full-body weight-training program, combined with a diet, puts you in the driver's seat on the path to positive changes.

Weight training changes your appearance. It also changes the way you feel about yourself by creating a positive self-image. You are in control of the way you look and feel. You control your health and happiness.

Your body's genetic blueprint modulates the range of change your body can undergo, but there is undoubtedly a great span between where you are now and what you can become. Hence, weight training provides you with the opportunity to redesign your body.

It's your body—take control of it through weight training. How you exercise that control will substantially influence your self-image.

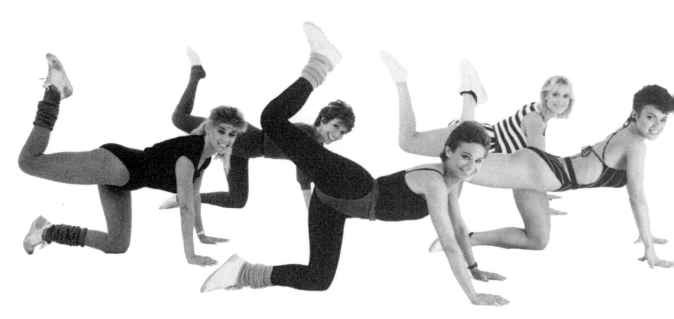

3
WEIGHT TRAINING'S PLACE IN FITNESS

School, kindergarten through college, is of little practical value if what's learned has no "real life" application. The same can be said of fitness programs. Which leads to these questions: What are the real life applications of a fitness program? What are the practical rewards of running, lifting, stretching, and dieting?

Fitness is an elusive term. Fit for what? Fit to mow the lawn? Fit to play tennis on the weekend? Fit to pass a series of fitness tests?

Exercise scientists, trying to carve a vocational niche, establish performance baselines in an attempt to quantify "fitness." For example, if one can elevate his or her heart rate above a certain level for a given amount of time, he or she is pronounced "aerobically fit." The connection between training guidelines and practical rewards is often neglected.

There *are* practical rewards, however, and we'll focus on these in this chapter. In addition to looking great, there are many other benefits derived from a weight-training program. First, let's review the components of fitness as defined by the American College of Sports Medicine, the country's largest organization of fitness professionals. Those components are:

- Muscular strength
- Aerobic endurance
- Muscular endurance
- Flexibility
- Body composition

Weight training has a demonstrably positive impact on four of the five above-listed fitness components. By comparison, distance running positively impacts only three. But we're running ahead of the story. Let's backtrack, explaining the impact of weight training on the five fitness components.

FITNESS COMPONENT: STRENGTH

Muscular strength is the greatest force the muscles can produce in a single effort. It refers to the force of a *single* maximum push, heave, or pull. The ACSM recommends weight training to satisfy "a need for a well-rounded program that exercises all the major muscle groups of the body."

Increased strength makes many of life's physical activities easier, including everything from running up a flight of stairs to twisting the cap off a resistant jelly jar. There is also a direct connection between increased strength and increased muscular endurance.

Real physical changes occur in the muscle cell when strength increases. The most noticeable is that the muscle cell increases in size by increasing the number of force-generating "bands" that run the length of the muscle cell. That's the basis of body sculpting, a "sidebar" to the fitness applications of weight training.

Just remember, muscular strength is the greatest force the muscle can produce in a single effort. And weight training is a proven path to quick strength gains.

FITNESS COMPONENT: MUSCULAR ENDURANCE

Muscular endurance is quite different from muscular strength. Whereas muscular strength is the measure of a single maximum effort, muscular endurance is the measure of the number of repetitions a muscle can perform against a fixed resistance.

There is a definite relationship between muscular endurance and strength. For example, let's say Jane can manage a single bench-press movement with 100 pounds, while George can perform a single bench press with 50 pounds. If both Jane and George use 25 pounds, Jane will be able to perform many more repetitions than George. Greater strength has given Jane a practical advantage in muscular endurance.

The muscular strength-endurance connection is the primary reason men have an advantage over women in competitions dependent on muscular endurance. Because the typical male develops greater strength than the typical female, it follows that the man can achieve greater measurable muscular endurance.

Muscular-endurance training has little practical application to everyday activities. You need turn the stuck jelly jar cap but once each morning. Hence, it makes little sense to gear a training program toward improving muscular endurance.

Although high-rep weight training can improve muscular endurance too, it's probably a waste of your time. Your weight-training time is better spent performing sets of 10 repetitions. Those sets will build strength and sculpt the body.

FITNESS COMPONENT: AEROBIC ENDURANCE

The fitness buff's main goal throughout aerobic training is to increase the body's ability to boost energy production by increasing oxygen delivery to working muscles. That's because energy production in the muscle is more efficient with oxygen than without oxygen.

A trained muscle can feed on itself for energy for about two minutes without the help of oxygen. But for longer periods of exertion, the muscle must rely on oxygen sent by the heart and lungs, delivered via the blood, and "burned" within the muscle.

Continuous activity for twenty to thirty minutes that elevates the heart rate to its "training zone" is the recommended method of improving oxygen-delivery capacity. That activity might be running, swimming, cycling, aerobic dancing, or any other activity that elevates the heart rate to its training zone and keeps it there for twenty to thirty minutes. This doesn't happen during weight training.

An appropriate training zone is different for each of us, but a rough calculation of the training zone is a simple task. Here's how it's done. Step one is to subtract your age from 220. The second step is to multiply the resulting number by 60 percent and 90 percent. Your training zone, the heart rate you should achieve during exercise, is the range of numbers falling between the high and low.

Let's use a thirty-year-old weight trainer as an example for determining a training zone.

$$\text{Step One: } 220 - 30 = 190$$
$$\text{Step Two: } 190 \times 60\% = 114$$
$$\text{and } 190 \times 90\% = 171$$

The training zone is between 114 and 171 beats per minute.

Frankly, weight training is not the best fitness activity for improving aerobic fitness. An appropriately high heart rate isn't maintained during a typical sequence of weight-training exercises. On the other hand, weight training does satisfy the training guidelines for the four remaining fitness components.

The best advice: cross-train. Combine weight training with an aerobic activity for complete fitness. More about this later in the chapter.

FITNESS COMPONENT: FLEXIBILITY

Flexibility is often taken for granted. But like strength or endurance, it is considered an integral component of complete fitness—and it can be improved through training.

Flexibility is the ability of the joints, muscles, and connective tissue that connect those joints to move through a full range of motion. For example, a flexible elbow is able to fully straighten or fully bend so that the hand touches the shoulder.

Weight-training exercises increase flexibility by lengthening the muscles. The more flexible muscle is less likely to be injured during a cross-training cardiovascular endurance activity like swimming or racquetball.

Flexibility also has practical applications in leisure-time activities. The golfer with a full range of motion in the torso and shoulders will execute a better swing. The skier will take fewer spills as her more flexible hip rotators and leg muscles enhance agility and rhythm. And greater flexibility increases the ease with which you might bend down to tie your shoes.

Weight training offers a triple whammy of fitness benefits: strength, muscular endurance, and flexibility.

FITNESS COMPONENT: BODY COMPOSITION

Body composition refers to the ratio of fat tissue to muscle tissue. "Leanness" is the related goal.

Weight training builds muscle tissue. A calorie-restricted diet can reduce fat. The combination of weight training and diet provides a double whammy toward a leaner body.

The typical American male carries about 20 percent of his body weight as fat. The typical American female carries a little more, about 25 percent. As important as physical health, body composition influences how we feel about ourselves: Are we fit or fat?

Body fat is not all bad. In fact, too little body fat is a health risk. Fats act as internal padding, which is vital for protecting internal organs from impact damage. And fat is the main source of energy storage for the body—when fat is exhausted, muscle is detroyed to produce needed energy.

Of course, too much body fat can be a health risk, too. But that's not always the case: There are people with body-fat percentages greater than 50 percent who are still fit and healthy. Most people who weight train, however, are usually more inclined to follow the cultural trend toward a thin, muscular look.

Weight training or any other exercise regimen won't change your fat-muscle ratio if you give no attention to diet too. Calories must be counted. You can burn a thousand extra calories exercising and still increase your body fat if you eat an additional eleven hundred calories. Conversely, you can forget exercise and eat less and improve your body composition—chronic dieters do it all the time. The point is moderation—exercise and diet in moderation to safely restructure body composition.

The best advice for a stronger, healthier, leaner body is to combine weight training and a calorie-restricted diet. You'll feel good and you'll look good.

We've now reviewed the five most frequently recognized fitness components. Notice that they're all *physical* components. The ACSM guidelines treat the psychological benefits of fitness as an afterthought. But self-image is often the primary reason for beginning a fitness program.

How we feel about ourselves is often the most important result of a fitness program. Fitness is a positive self-esteem builder. That's the case whether it's bigger biceps or a lower pulse rate that precipitates the feelings. Having said that, it's time to move on to more about physical fitness.

The best way to acquire and maintain ultimate physical fitness is through cross-training.

COMBINING WEIGHT TRAINING AND AEROBICS

When the first edition of this book was published in 1978, the term *cross-training* hadn't been coined. But weight trainers who ran were doing it anyway.

The running boom of the early 1970s indirectly bred the cross-training boom. Large numbers of runners, many taking it to an extreme, stimulated a popular discussion of the meaning of fitness. Running upward of fifty miles a week allowed runners to build great aerobic endurance, but often produced "bone-racks." You still see these skin-covered skeletons winning international marathon events. Is that fitness?

Less obsessive runners—not wanting to go the way of the bone-racks—chose a more moderate program: three miles, three days a week. They turned to weight training as a supplement to running. Combining weight training and running produced aerobic fitness while maintaining a pleasing physique. The combination produced a broader spectrum of benefits than could be had through either activity practiced alone.

The conclusion reached was that complete fitness meant more than being just aerobically fit. Soon, the five ACSM guidelines evolved into the benchmarks of fitness. Since no one activity is best for all five components, cross-training evolved. The most popular form of cross-training is combining weight training with an aerobic activity. Let's explore several examples.

Combining Weight Training and Aerobic Dance

Weight training combined with aerobic dance or step-aerobics provides an excellent fitness package. Additionally, you can easily perform this training within the privacy and space limitations of a home gym. This cross-training combination improves and maintains all five fitness components.

Mixing and matching movements and training stresses from both activities offers a condensed, yet complete, workout. For example, twenty minutes of a step workout will enhance aerobic fitness while strengthening and firming the legs and hips. Following the step-aerobics with weight training strengthens and shapes the upper body—an area little affected by the step workout.

Weight train and step on the same day, or split your routine by stepping one day and lifting the next. However your time constraints dictate your schedule, step three days a week and lift three days a week.

Combining Dumbbells with Your Favorite Step Bench Movements

Using dumbbells with step bench movements is very popular in health club aerobics classes, and it's an activity you can perform at home. It's a fun, challenging, time-saving complete workout.

The rationale is this: Stepping strengthens the lower body musculature as well as the cardiovascular system, while the dumbbells strengthen the upper body.

With a little bit of practice, you can coordinate the arm and step movements. Once you've mastered several basic step movements with your legs, adding dumbbell exercises for your arms and shoulders are a snap. I recommend dumbbell presses (p. 153), bicep curls (p. 118), and upright rows (p. 158)—demonstrated in the photo below. Start

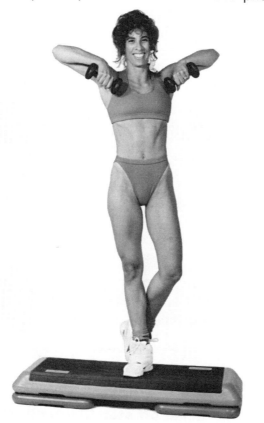

Step Bench with Weights

with lighter weights (two to five pounds) than you would use for stationary exercises. It will take a little practice to control that extra resistance at the end of your arms while moving your legs.

Carey Filbert, an aerobics instructor and fitness consultant, believes that the combo weight-step bench workout effectively works the biceps, triceps, the shoulders, hips, and legs. She advises that the typical weight-step bench routine be "supplemented with non-step free weight exercises for the chest, back, and abdominals. These muscle groups aren't effectively exercised with an erect, stepping posture." Supplemental exercises such as resistance push-ups (pp. 128–132), chest flys (p. 136), and bent-over rows (p. 117) will complete the workout.

Like other fitness activities, a warm-up and cool down stretch is incorporated into a weight-step bench workout to target the muscles used. For example, stretch-lunges off the step platform loosen the leg muscles prior to the more demanding step routine (see photo).

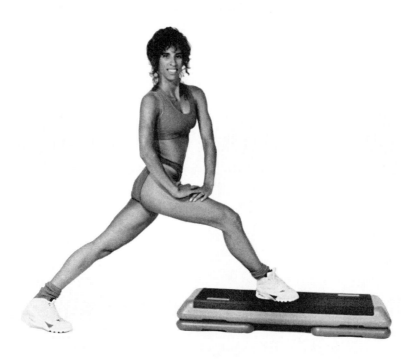

Lunge off step bench platform

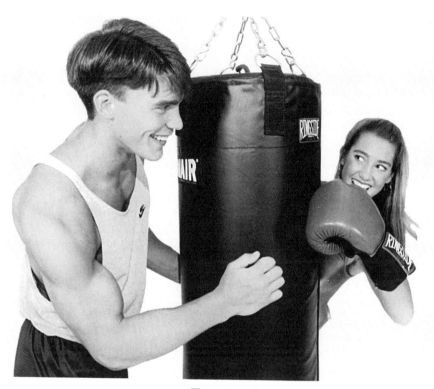

Two boxing partners and heavy bag

Combining Weight Training and Boxing

Weight training and boxing? Boxers are among the best conditioned of athletes. You might not want the lumps, bumps, and cuts boxers endure, but you can borrow the heavy bag and jump rope from a boxer's repertoire to supplement your weight-training routine.

Pounding the heavy bag builds upper-body muscular endurance. Punching requires continual use of the arms, shoulders, chest, and rotational muscles of your torso. The jump rope builds lower-body muscular endurance. Alternating between the bag (three minutes) and the rope (two minutes) for twenty continuous minutes also provides an intense aerobic workout.

If you've never hit a heavy bag before, try hitting it 30 beats per minute with low to moderate force. Alternate punches, left, right, left, right. Stand six inches short of arm's length from the bag so that your punch pushes the bag at the full extension of the arm. As your condition improves, gradually increase the tempo and the force. Always take care not to turn your wrists when learning to hit a heavy bag. You can do this by concentrating on maintaining a straight line between the back of your hand and the forearm as you strike the bag.

Rope skipping develops stamina, speedy footwork, and it limbers up the arms, wrists and shoulders. After mastering the standard form of jumping, improvise your footwork and rope movements. Try reversing the rope as you jump, or bring the rope around for two revolutions between each landing (double loop). The main point is that you continuously move your arms and legs during the two minutes. The style is your choice; make it fun.

An intense aerobic workout can be had from alternating between the bag and the rope. Punch the bag for three minutes. Then jump rope in place for two minutes. Return to punching for three and jumping for two and so on until the twenty minutes are up. Combining weights with the boxer's repertoire will provide an effective, exhaustive fifty minutes, that breaks down into twenty minutes on the bag and rope and thirty minutes of weight training.

One final note concerning the bag. Purchase a water bag—no joke—a water bag. There are several manufacturers of punching bags that use water rather than batten to fill the bag. The water bag has a practical advantage: The shock of the punch is more slowly absorbed by the water bag, lessening the jar to your wrists and elbows.

Combining the bag, rope, and weight training makes for an enjoyable, complete fitness workout, one that can be performed in the corner of your garage or basement.

COMBINING WEIGHTS WITH A SKI MACHINE, OR EXERCYCLE, OR STAIR CLIMBER MACHINE

The popularity of ski machines, exercise bikes, and stair climber machines is justified by their ability to deliver a good aerobic workout. Keep in mind, though, that none of these mechanical devices adequately exercises and strengthens every important muscle group.

The primary drawback is that each machine limits the number of potential movements, thereby limiting the number of muscles involved in the workout. For example, the muscles responsible for raising the arms above the head aren't being adequately exercised on a ski machine or exercycle.

I find that combining a standard weight workout for strength build-

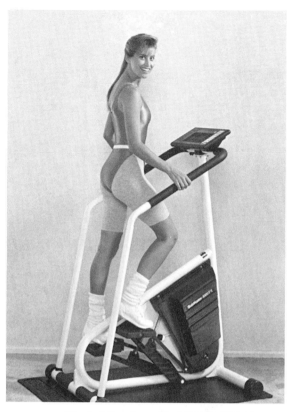

StairMaster ™ 4000 PT ® exercise system

ing with the StairMaster 4000 PT for increasing aerobic capacity effectively works a full parcel of fitness components.

You can combine weight training with any of the aerobic-fitness machines for a complete workout. It's a matter of personal choice.

Cross-training your way to complete fitness is as easy as combining weight training with any of the activities featured in this chapter. Of course, you can combine weight training with all of them at various times of the year—all in the privacy and space limitations of your home gym.

There are many other activities, such as swimming, running, or racquetball, if you prefer getting out of the house. But the formula for complete fitness remains the same regardless of environmental preference: The combination of weight training and an aerobic activity delivers all five fitness components.

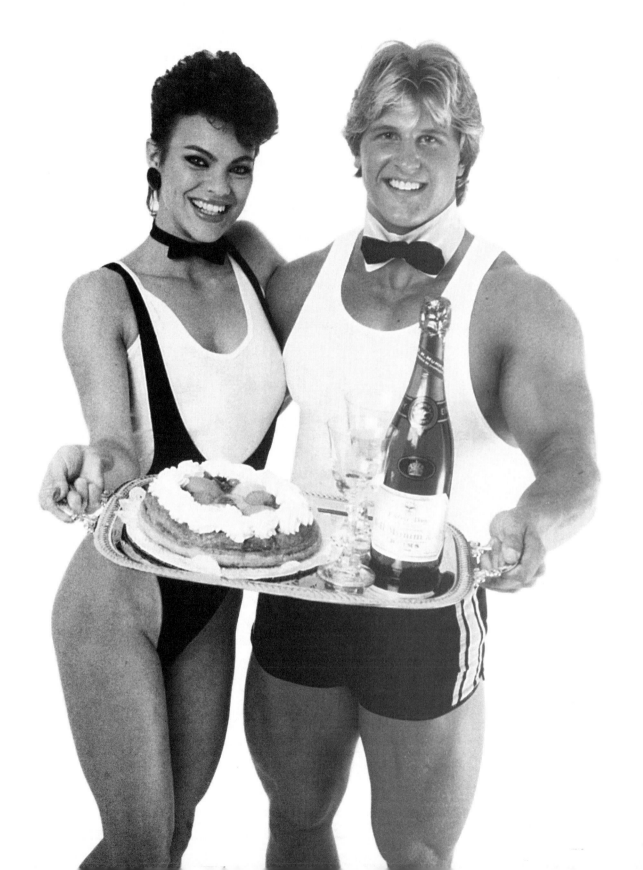

4
NUTRITION: YOU ARE WHAT YOU EAT

The saying "You are what you eat" is at least metaphorically correct. That's why some people look like too many jelly doughnuts. What you eat also partly defines what you are able to do. That's why your goal as a weight trainer is to select foods that enhance your training program, combining exercise and diet to build a stronger, healthier, more attractive body.

Selecting the right foods need not be complicated. All the foods that we eat—Hershey's Kisses to an apple to a salad—can be arranged into six groups, each of which has special qualities that satisfy different body needs. Those six groups—liquids, proteins, fats, carbohydrates, vitamins, and minerals—are collectively called "basic nutrients."

The U.S. Department of Agriculture recommends that those nutrients be obtained through a daily diet of:

- six to eleven servings from the pasta, bread, cereal, and rice group;
- three to five servings of vegetables;
- two to four servings of fruits;
- two to three servings from the milk, yogurt, and cheese group; and
- two to three servings from the meat, poultry, fish, dry beans, eggs, and nuts group;

A REVIEW OF THE BASIC NUTRIENTS

The six groups perform only three jobs. They supply energy, act as building blocks for tissue growth or repair, and act as catalysts in the body's thousands of life-supporting reactions.

Some of the nutrients do several different jobs. For example, protein is the primary building block of muscle tissue, but can also be tapped as an energy source.

The following is an overview of the basic groups and examples of how they interact with your training program.

Minerals

Minerals needed to keep your body healthy and strong—iron, chromium, potassium, copper, and so on—are the same ones taken from the ground and used to manufacture the iron barbells and chrome-plated machines that are part of your training program.

Minerals are a natural part of the food that we eat. Plants growing in mineral-rich soils absorb minerals into their roots, stems, leaves, and fruit. Then we eat the plants or eat animals that have eaten the plants. That's why whole grains, fruit, milk, and vegetables provide the best supply of essential minerals.

Where minerals originate is one thing; how the body utuilizes them is another. Iron is an excellent example of how a mineral interacts with our training program. Iron is the primary building block of hemoglobin, a chemical compound that carries oxygen along our bloodstream.

Once in the lungs, oxygen catches a ride on hemoglobin to each living cell throughout our bodies. In the cell, oxygen interacts with foodstuffs to release energy. Without the hemoblogin-building iron, not enough oxygen would reach our cells to meet the energy demands of training.

No less important than its role in oxygen delivery, the iron-rich hemoglobin also carries carbon dioxide, a harmful by-product of energy production, from the cell to the lung. Once in the lung, the harmful carbon dioxide is expelled from the body.

Including iron, your body needs sixteen different minerals in varying amounts. A lack of only one of the sixteen minerals can severely harm your body. That's why it's important to include mineral-rich foods as part of your overall diet. Not only will your training suffer, but your health is at risk with a diet containing inadequate minerals.

Eat those vegetables.

Vitamins

All foods contain vitamins. But like minerals, they are not found in adequate amounts in a single food. That's why it's important for the weight trainer to eat a wide selection of foods—the so-called "well-balanced diet."

Unlike our example of the mineral iron, vitamins don't directly contribute to the structure of the body's tissues. Nor do they contain energy or calories as do fats, carbohydrates, and proteins. Nevertheless, they are essential contributors in all building, maintenance, and energy-producing processes.

Vitamins help absorb minerals, synthesize hormones, utilize proteins, and impact bone production. For example, vitamin C is necessary in hormone synthesis. Inadequate amounts of vitamin C in the diet could negatively impact the production of the hormones responsible for muscle growth and maintenance—an unnecessary handicap for any weight-training program. Vitamin C also improves the absorption of iron.

Vitamin D is essential for the body to absorb and utilize calcium and phosphorus. In fact, there's a direct connection between bones, calcium, phosphorus, vitamin D, and weight training.

Weight training increases the strength of bones. In fact, weight training is the best exercise for building stronger bones. How does this strength increase occur? Bones respond to the stress of weight training by packing on more bone-building materials, calcium, and phosphorus. The bones become thicker in cross-section and more densely packed as the calcium and phosphorus is added. The added minerals act on bone much as steel girders act to strengthen a bridge or building.

Without vitamin D in the diet, the body is prevented from adding bone as an adaptive response to weight training. In fact, a continuing deficiency of vitamin D induces atrophy of bone and connective tissue, increasing the likelihood of injury.

Vitamin D is an example of a fat-soluble vitamin, as are vitamins A, E, and K. A fat-soluble vitamin must combine with fats in order to carry out its duties, but missing a few days of a fat-soluble vitamin isn't likely to cause you many problems. That's because fat-soluble vitamins are stored in the body's fat. On the other hand, too much of a fat-soluble vitamin—because it is readily stored—creates a toxic effect, particularly in the liver. That's why weight trainers are best advised to stay away from high-dosage vitamin pills containing vitamins A, D, E, and K.

Water-soluble vitamins aren't stored; excessive amounts are flushed out with the urine. For that reason, water-soluble vitamins are a daily dietary necessity. Without an adequate supply, the weight trainer's performance is compromised. For example, a deficiency of B-complex vitamins degrades nerve impulses, produces muscular fatigue, induces cramps, and raises blood pressure. That's why it's advisable to take a daily vitamin pill containing water-soluble vitamins. Speaking of water, that's the next essential nutrient on our list.

Water

Water makes up over 70 percent of the weight of a muscle, as well as 60 percent of our total body weight. It has no vitamins, minerals, or usable energy, yet it is second to oxygen as the body's most needed substance. Only a 2-percent weight loss from dehydration (that's three pounds for a 150-pound weight trainer) raises the body temperature above 100 degrees Fahrenheit. Dehydration affects all body functions.

We satisfy most of our water needs through the liquids we drink, but our bodies also have another source of water. The solid foods we eat contain substantial amounts, from the 5-percent-water soda cracker, to the 90-percent-water stalk of celery.

The weight trainer should continually drink water or other liquids, even during workouts. Most training specialists recommend six to eight glasses of liquid a day. That six to eight glasses is all-inclusive, from diet drinks to coffee (remember, coffee is a diuretic). Whenever and whatever liquid is consumed, the best advice is to take small, frequent drinks. Large gulps will unnecessarily bloat the stomach, because the bloodstream can absorb only about a quart per hour.

Let the liquid flow.

Protein: Strings of Amino Acids

Proteins can be found in each of your body's cells. There are structural proteins, the so-called "building blocks," and there are other proteins that act as enzymes, or catalysts that speed up numerous biological reactions.

Proteins are made of long strings of small clumps of chemicals. Each clump along the string is called an amino acid. There are over twenty different kinds of amino acids. Those twenty different amino acids can be arranged along the string in thousands of different combinations. Each different combination is a different protein.

It might be easier for you to imagine proteins as strings of hundreds or thousands of beads, each bead having one of twenty colors. The order of the beads determines the type of protein.

The weight trainer needs all of the twenty-plus amino acids to maintain or build a healthy body, and that's the rub—not all foods contain proteins with all the amino acids. Sources of "complete proteins"— those with all the amino acids—are meat, eggs, and milk. Most plants have "incomplete proteins," lacking one or more of the amino acids.

A well-balanced diet contains all the necessary amino acids that you'll need. Amino acids lacking in one food are supplied by another. After the food-source protein chains are broken into amino acids during digestion, your body recombines those amino acids into new proteins that meet your human biological needs.

ENERGY FOODS: CARBOHYDRATES AND FATS

Carbohydrates and fats are the weight trainer's primary sources of food energy. Carbohydrates are much more quickly digested and turned into energy than are fats. On the other hand, fats have the highest concentration of energy of all foods: more than 4,200 calories per pound, compared to about 1,700 for carbohydrates.

After becoming part of the body, stored fat has an even greater energy advantage: 3,500 calories can be culled from a pound of fat, compared to 250 from a pound of stored carbohydrates. That means that fat is great news for energetic weight watchers: A week's supply of energy can be stored as six pounds of fat—or seventy pounds of carbohydrates.

Protein foodstuffs can also be used as a source of energy if the intake of fats and carbohydrates is insufficient. But we will not deal with protein as an energy source in the following material. The use of protein as a primary energy source implies an inappropriate diet for the weight trainer.

Carbohydrates

Carbohydrates are the main source of food energy for the weight trainer. Carbohydrates are essential in the daily diet, because most bodies store less than a pound and that doesn't go very far. For example, more than that is burned during a marathon.

Carbohydrates in our diet come from plants or from animals that eat plants. The earliest fossil record suggests that plants, through photosynthesis, were able to manufacture carbohydrates 3.5 billion years ago. The fossil record doesn't suggest that there were any animals present to eat them.

A primary energy source for animals today are carbohydrate-bearing plants. People have learned to cultivate these carbohydrates, such as wheats, grains, and cereals, that have become so common in our diet.

In 1991, Americans consumed 2.7 billion pounds of cereal, a 2,255-percent increase over 1990. Apparently, people are eating cereal around the clock.

Cereal with milk is a good source of calcium and pre- or posttraining carbohydrates. As a rule of thumb, avoid granolas, which can contain more than 30 percent fat. Special vitamin-fortified cereals are unnecessary when the rest of your food intake is balanced.

The carbohydrates in cereals and other foods that we eat are composed of sugar molecules. Three types of sugar molecules—glucose, fructose, and galactose—pass from the intestine into the bloodstream during digestion.

Glucose provides so-called "quick energy." That's because it passes more quickly from the intestine to the bloodstream and directly to the area of energy demand. Fructose and galactose must stop at the liver before moving on to the area of need. That's why eating honey or a candy bar provides quick energy, because they both contain natural glucose.

Muscles can't be maintained without an adequate supply of carbohydrates. Carbohydrates are integral to protein metabolism, and protein metabolism is essential to building and maintaining muscle tissue. Chances are that you won't even feel like training if you're deprived of carbohydrates, because the brain depends on glucose from your bloodstream for energy.

Eat a daily supply of carbohydrates.

Fats

All foods contain fat, ranging from 100 percent for lard to less than 1 percent in most fruits and vegetables. Fat in the diet is a necessary component for energy and health.

Most energy stored in the body is stored in the form of fat. But you don't have to eat fat in order to store it, because the excess carbohydrates and proteins that you eat can be converted and stored as fat.

Body fat has a bad reputation in our lean, mean culture. But a little stored fat is necessary for health and safety. Without fat, the body could not store or utilize fat-soluble vitamins. Fat also acts as safety pads around internal organs, while subcutaneous fat insulates us on those cold winter nights.

Fats are easily obtained in the diet. Cream, milk, cheese, butter, egg yolks, and meat have lots of fat. Maybe too much fat. Most nutritionists recommend that the athlete receive 20 to 25 percent of daily calorie consumption from fat. More about that in the next section of this chapter.

WEIGHT TRAINER'S GENERAL GUIDELINES

Foods supply energy and essential nutrients. The weight trainer's goal is to choose foods that meet the body's total energy needs while supplying the necessary amounts of essential nutrients.

Total energy needs depend on the body's activity level. All foods contain energy, but the balance between energy consumption and energy use determines whether you're eating the right amount. It's easy enough to step on a scale to determine if you're consuming too much or too little energy.

Consume more energy than your activity level demands and you'll gain weight. Consume less energy than your activity level demands and you'll lose weight. Match consumption with needs and your weight will remain stable. As a practical matter, that's all you need know about the relationship between energy consumption, activity level, and body weight.

A more precise method of tabulating your energy consumption is counting calories. A calorie is a unit measure of energy. If you feel more comfortable with the precision of counting calories than relying on a scale, purchase a booklet that lists the calorie content of common foods. They're often available from the rack at the supermarket checkout line.

Since energy is available from all foods, it is conceivable that 100 percent of your energy demands could be met from only one food—perhaps a scoop of lard or pound after pound of string beans. But research and practical observation overwhelmingly support the conclusion that a diverse diet is a healthier diet. A healthy combination of diverse foods is the so-called "well-balanced diet."

The weight trainer's well-balanced diet is one in which the foods he or she eats contains 60 percent carbohydrates, 25 percent fats, and 15 percent proteins. That mix of carbohydrates, fats, and proteins should be derived from a broad selection of fruits, vegetables, grains, dairy products, and meats so that all the body's essential vitamins, minerals, and amino acids are supplied. That's a nutshell explanation of a well-balanced diet.

The weight trainer's diet is no different from that recommended to the average person. Of course, when compared with a less active person, the added activity of weight training begets greater energy demands, and requires more food. But the 60-25-15 ratio remains the same within the new energy parameters.

The best advice is simple. Eat a well-balanced diet with the recommended percentages of carbohydrates, fats, and proteins. As a safety precaution, swallow a moderate-dosage pill of minerals and water-soluble vitamins. Drink six to eight glasses of liquid a day.

Couple that diet with regular training and you're on your way to a stronger, healthier, more attractive body. Let's ask and answer related questions to drive the message home.

Should I eat more when weight training?

Weight training is not a big energy consumer. The precise energy expenditure during a typical weight-training workout depends on exercise selection, poundages lifted, and the size of the weight trainer.

An "average" weight trainer expends less than 500 calories during a workout. That's equivalent to the calories provided by a cheeseburger. Hence, there's really nothing special about the energy demands of weight training.

Are vitamin and mineral supplements needed when weight training?

No. A well-balanced diet provides the vitamins and minerals necessary for general health and a successful weight-training program.

However, as an insurance policy for those of you concerned about eating a well-balanced diet—studies indicate that about half of you don't—a multivitamin and mineral tablet is a good idea. Don't consume megadoses of any vitamin or mineral, particularly megadoses of fat-soluble vitamins (A, D, E and K). The fat-solubles can accumulate in your body's tissue and produce toxic side effects.

Do weight trainers need extra protein?

Weight trainers need no greater supply of protein than any other person of similar size and weight.

During the 1970s, weight trainers and bodybuilders ate enormous quantities of protein, thinking it necessary to build strength and muscle. Some of those old-time lifters ate as much as five pounds of meat each day, until the unbalanced diet led to health problems. The moral of the story is that gorging your body with extra protein doesn't help but could hurt.

How much protein is both adequate and safe?

One-half gram of protein per day for each pound of body weight is a good rule of thumb. That means that 75 grams of protein needs to be in each day's food supply for a 150-pound weight trainer. That much protein can be found in a chicken leg, two eggs, and two cups of milk.

Do I need protein and amino-acid supplements?

A weight trainer who eats a well-balanced diet doesn't need a protein and amino-acid supplement. It's just money down the drain. If you feel you need more protein, just eat more high-protein foods.

DIETING WHILE WEIGHT TRAINING

Moderate calorie reduction to lose a few pounds and create a more defined look is not devastating to the weight trainer's body, but extreme calorie-deficient diets can devastate a weight trainer's performance.

Let's imagine a weight trainer with an energy expenditure of 4,700 calories a day. He consumes 4,200 calories, a 500-calorie deficit over expenditure. How can that weight trainer expend 500 calories more than he consumes?

That extra 500 calories of energy has to come from somewhere, so his body feeds on itself. There's a cannibal inside each of us.

How does it work? After the body has exploited the energy from recently eaten food, it taps stores of fat and glycogen. If the stored fat and glycogen are completely depleted through extended dieting, the body will then feed on its own protein—the protein that the weight trainer needs to build and repair muscle.

Practical advice for the weight trainer on a diet is to limit daily calorie intake to no less than 400 calories below energy expenditures. The weight trainer must be sure to keep the balance of nutrients such that protein intake meets the body's needs. Cut fats to cut calories.

A final note. You can't grow bigger muscles while on a weight-loss diet. In short, the body won't support new growth while having to feed on itself for energy.

Can I spot reduce by dieting and weight training?

Spot reducing is absolutely not possible through weight training. A thousand situps a day for six months won't remove an inch off your stomach: spot reducing doesn't work. The exercise will, however, firm and tone the muscles of the stomach. But removing inches of fat requires eating fewer calories.

In conclusion, the weight trainer can relax, count calories, and eat a well-balanced diet. For security, swallow a multivitamin-mineral tablet once a day.

You'll still be besieged by the latest nutritional fads in magazines and on TV, but consider the following quote before jumping on any unproven bandwagons:

> "When you go into a health-food store, it's like being the victim of a hundred different snake-oil salesmen. The public needs some protection in this jungle of a marketplace."
>
> —Michael Jacobson, 1993
> Center for Science in the Public Interest

Don't be a victim. All that's necessary to be successful in your weight-training program is to eat a well-balanced diet and train hard.

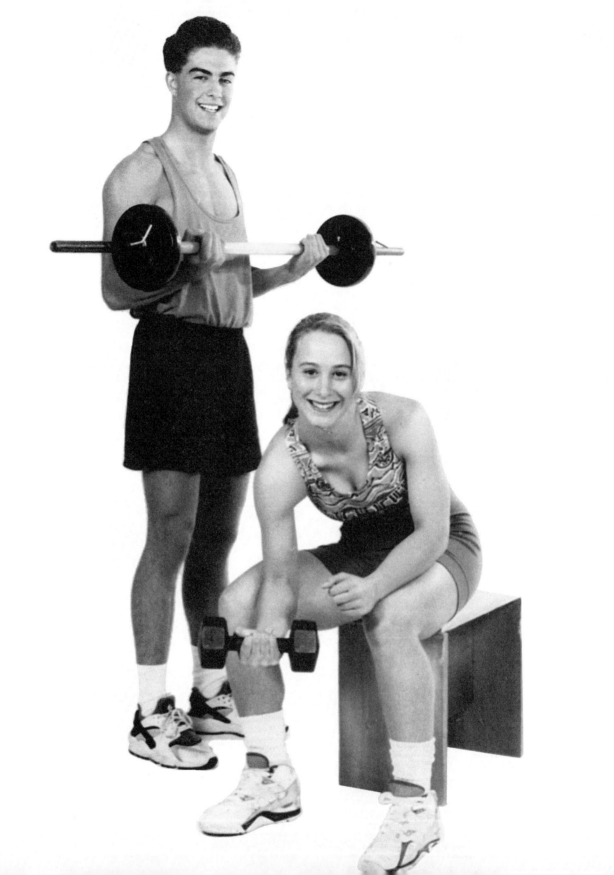

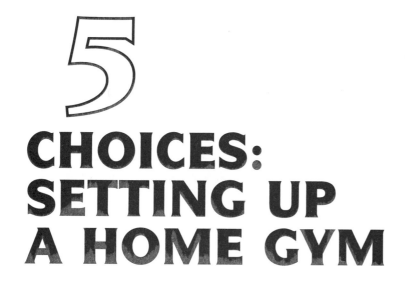

5

CHOICES: SETTING UP A HOME GYM

Once having made the decision to weight train, the next choice is where to weight train. Home gym or commercial facility? Consider your financial investment: Should you take your annual health-club dues and invest in a home gym?

Each has advantages. A home gym offers absolute control, convenience, and the elimination of travel time to and from the gym. You can do things your way, any time you choose. But a home gym can't match the range of equipment and amenities offered by a modern commercial facility, or the aura of the mecca, Gold's Gym. To be sure, there are trade-offs, but a great workout can be had at either place.

Like millions of other weight trainers, let's assume you too have made the decision to train at home. Here's what to consider.

SPACE NEEDS

Weight training takes space. A separate, permanent space. Before shopping for equipment, designate a specific space. A special space contributes to commitment, which, in turn, enhances your workout.

You don't need a big space. An eight-by-twelve-foot area (spare room, basement area, or corner of the garage) will permanently house your equipment and provide ample space for the exercise routines recommended in this book.

Be sure to check the headroom, too. An eight-foot ceiling height accommodates all but the very tallest of weight trainers during overhead lifts.

Select a well-ventilated, well-lit space. Add the warmth of carpet and the "life" of a mirror if your budget permits. A mirror is a practical addition, offering visual feedback on exercise technique. A music system enhances a workout, inspiring you to make that last rep.

One final note on selecting a space. Before buying that first piece of equipment, use masking tape to outline appropriate places on the floor. Check door and hallway dimensions, too, to be sure that the equipment can reach the intended training area.

EQUIPMENT RECOMMENDATIONS

Free Weights

Barbells and dumbbells are so-called "free weights." They are so named because they allow freedom of movement, not because they're giveaways at your local sporting goods store.

Free weights are the focus of this book for two reasons. First, free weights are the least expensive and most common weight-training devices in the marketplace. The price of a beginning set of free weights costs about the same as a pair of medium-priced basketball shoes. The cast-iron weights will last forever and fit every member of the family, too. That's a bargain.

Second, free weights are appropriate for any body size. Most popular weight-training machines aren't. Most machines are designed for the average adult, leaving the tall and short of us in the lurch. An improper fit can compromise safety as well as minimize the intended effect of an exercise movement.

Expensive machines manufactured by Cybex, Flex, Nautilus, and others that lure customers into commercial gymnasiums use the same muscle-building principles as a hand-me-down set of barbells. The training intensity, not the cost of the equipment, determines the success of a weight-training program.

Barbells and dumbbells, so-called free weights, are tried and true weight-training equipment. There's no need to purchase expensive macines and gadgets. Will strength and size increase more quickly with machines? No.

This is not to imply that all machines are badly designed. But free weights have no "fit" problem, and they won't strain your wallet. Unlike most weight-training machines, a set of free weights will effectively exercise all muscle groups.

Olympic or Standard Plates?

You'll find two types of free weight systems, *standard* and *Olympic,* at your local sporting goods outlet. The difference between the two systems is the diameter of the bar and the hole size of the corresponding plates. I recommend the standard system. It's more readily adaptable for use as dumbbells. Also, the standard bar (without plates) weighs less than the plateless Olympic bar. The lighter bar provides the potential for a lower starting point for weaker lifters.

Most sporting goods stores offer different packages of free weights—combinations of 100 to 300 pounds of bars and plates. Pound for pound, the 300-pound set is most economical, but if you decide on a smaller starting set, you can always buy additional barbell plates when needed.

To reiterate, the standard set is the best to follow the exercises outlined in this book.

Don't Improvise Weights

Improvising weights to cut cost is also a mistake. Incorporating household devices by filling plastic jugs with sand and water might seem an expedient thing to do, but in practice, these objects are hard to balance, nearly impossible to calibrate, and difficult to grip.

Treat yourself to a safe, inexpensive set of free weights and set a serious tone to your weight-training program.

The Bench

The weight-training bench pictured in the exercise photos throughout this book has a bench-press support to cradle a barbell. The backrest can be adjusted to accommodate both flat and incline bench presses.

Benches come in all price ranges. The bench pictured herein can cost as little as $20 at a sporting goods store that sells used items. Fancier models can cost as much as a few hundred dollars.

Take care in selecting the bench. Buy one with bench-press supports. Don't buy on price alone. Remember that there will be times when you're lying on that bench with a heavy weight supported above your head. Check the welds. Check the general stability and fit by lying on a showroom model. Check the width, padding, and upholstery for comfort. Don't come home with what amounts to a torture rack.

Chin-Dip Bar

The chin-dip bar combination costs about $125 but is an invaluable piece of training equipment. (The model pictured in this book was purchased on sale at a retail sporting goods store for $99.) That one piece of equipment is a vehicle to exercising the musculature of the entire upper body.

The chin-dip bar is a sound investment. Without it, you are left avoiding certain exercises, or you're left to improvise with household appliances and furniture as chin-dip bars.

Those are your heavy equipment needs. Just three items: a barbell-dumbbell set, a bench, and a chin-dip bar combination.

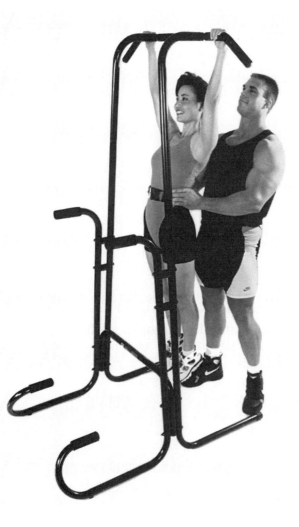

MACHINE SHOPPING TIPS

If you just can't resist, there are many home-gym machines from which to choose. The multistation units are popular and range anywhere from $400 to $1,500. What should you consider in making a decision to purchase?

1. **Assembly** is time-consuming and could produce unstable equipment. Does the unit shake and rattle during use, or is it sturdy and durable?
2. **Maximum resistance** is different on each machine. Will the resistance of a particular machine be enough as your body becomes stronger?
3. **Range of motion**: Does the machine permit a full range of motion during the intended exercise movement?
4. **Does it fit your body?** Are the seats the right height? Are the backrests the right width? Bench too narrow or too wide? Does it fit every body intending to use it?
5. **Full-body workout capacity?** Does the machine have attachments to work every major muscle group?
6. **Will it fit into your house?** Weight of unit, height, width, length?
7. **Motivationally deficient?** Does the machine require constant modification during a workout that produces annoying interruptions?

If in doubt about the efficacy of a particular machine, stick to your trusty set of free weights and spare yourself a potentially bad investment.

APPAREL AND ACCESSORIES

There was a time when one pair of sneakers would do for all your recreational activities. Since the writing of the first edition of this book fifteen years ago, there has been a revolution in the sports shoe and apparel industry. All categories of exercise clothing and shoes have become big business. According to the National Sporting Goods Association, $29 billion of sports equipment, gear, and clothing was sold in 1990.

Fashionable, high-tech, high-performance, scientifically designed gear promise to minimize injuries while providing a competitive edge, but for a price. What's necessary for weight training?

Training Clothes

When weight training vigorously, your muscles put out energy at the same rate as a 400-watt light bulb. About 70 percent of that energy output is heat energy. If that heat isn't somehow removed from the body, the average body's temperature would rise about six degrees in an hour.

The clothing you wear is an important factor in helping or hindering the removal of that heat. The blood moves the heat from the muscle to the skin, where the heat is transferred to sweat. At this point the heated sweat evaporates, carrying the heat into the atmosphere— unless clothing prevents that evaporation.

Loose-fitting clothes interact best with the body's natural cooling system. Tight clothing, especially rubberized garments, prevent air circulation at the surface of your skin. The sweat vapor is trapped near the skin, preventing further evaporation. The body's cooling system is effectively blocked.

Loose-fitting clothing is particularly important in humid weather. The body can endure dry heat of 200 degrees Fahrenheit for several hours and the cooling system keeps humming along. But when humidity is high, the evaporative process is partially blocked and the heated sweat remains on the skin.

Bare skin is best for the body's cooling system; millions of years of evolution saw to that. You can follow along with the recent clothing fad; just make sure garments are loose-fitting if you cover large areas of the body in warm, humid weather.

Training in cold weather can cause problems too. An internal temperature that's too low constricts the muscles' blood vessels. The excess blood needed to safely perform an exercise movement leaves the muscles to heat the core of the body. The warm blood exiting the muscle increases the potential for injury to the muscle and associated joints.

Unlike warm-weather training, it's best to cover up in cold weather to retain the body's heat.

Shoes, Gloves, and Belts

For the weight trainer, training shoes and lifting gloves are available at any sporting goods store. Both are a wise and important investment.

Weight training requires a shoe with firm sole and arch support, and a flexible top. Basketball shoes fit the bill. So do aerobic dance shoes and cross-training shoes. All have the lateral support necessary for safe execution of many weight-training exercises. Running shoes are usually not good for weight training, since they're designed for a limited range of use—forward motion.

Gloves are especially practical for beginners. The friction of the barbell or dumbbells interacting with unconditioned skin has caused many a blister. Gloves are inexpensive, and will guard against workout interruptions due to sore hands. They will also ensure adequate grip.

Lifting belts are a matter of personal choice. I have never worn a lifting belt through thirty-five years of weight-training experience. However, I've known many experienced weight trainers who recommend using a belt anytime the exercise involves use of the lower back. I have found no research to indicate that belts do, in fact, prevent injuries or improve performance, but it's intuitively reasonable that the support provided by the belt adds a level of safety to an exercise involving the lower back.

TRAINING PARTNERS

Training partners help, especially at home, and they don't just help by lifting a weight off of you when you're stuck. They add inspiration to a workout, count reps, monitor form, act as a natural rest break by alternating exercises, and sometimes they help simply by dragging you into the gym on a day when your motivation is low.

Training partners come in all ages, shapes, sizes, and genders. Enlist friends, family, or gym buddies. The training partner adds safety, camaraderie, and motivation to a workout.

Sometimes the training partner takes on the hat of supervisor, especially if the weight trainer is a beginner, child, or adolescent. In fact, the American Academy of Pediatrics, and most other researchers, recommend supervision by trained adults when children and adolescents engage in a strength-training program.

Experience level and age aside, a primary responsibility of a training partner is to spot during many exercises. That brings to mind an important point: The training partner must be fit for the job.

Spotters—Even at Home

Certain lifts require spotters. A spotter assists, as needed, in the safe execution of the exercise. General guidelines for safe and effective spotting are:

- Know the correct form and the most likely points of failure during the exercise you're spotting.
- Secure the exercise location, removing any obstacle, such as loose barbell plates, that might interfere with your spotting.
- Check that the collars are tight.
- Before the exercise begins, establish with the lifter the point at which you will assist, and the number of intended reps.
- Place your body in a "ready position," knees flexed and hands close to the bar throughout the exercise movement.
- Be sure that you can support the entire weight if necessary. If not, *you* need an assistant.

If you're a spotter, and unsure of your ability to spot a given exercise, don't do it. Both you and the lifter could be hurt. Advise the lifter to find another spotter or skip the lift.

PERSONAL TRAINERS: A PERSONAL FIT

Amid busy schedules and numerous obligations, more and more men and women are turning to personal trainers to maximize their workout time or provide an informed introduction to weight training. A personal trainer can meet you at home or at the gym.

A knowledgeable personal trainer can customize a weight-training routine to match your specific goal, whether it is improved strength, shape, cardiovascular endurance, or a combination of fitness factors. Before you get started, expect to first share background information with your trainer, who may ask for a complete health history and lifestyle assessment in order to design an individualized training program and dietary regimen. Personal trainers also provide the motivation that might otherwise be lacking.

Motivation is no small contribution. While you might have run out of steam on your own, a trainer keeps the pace going *without* overdoing it. An hour of personalized, quality training is the end result.

Most health clubs (and hotels if you're traveling) will provide a list of personal trainers. You can find a personal trainer to work according to your schedule.

If you're brand new to weight training and you have no training partner, plan on having the personal trainer stay with you for the first half-dozen workouts. Once you've increased your knowledge of proper form and training sequence, you can decrease the number of one-on-one sessions. The personal trainer can always be brought in for occasional evaluations and corresponding restructuring of your workout schedule.

The fees of a personal trainer range from very affordable to steep. Some cost as little as $15 an hour, and some go up to $200 a half-hour session for a movie celebrity with a special look in mind. As with most services, the price is negotiable.

Over fifteen organizations now certify personal trainers. I recommend those certified through the American College of Sports Medicine or the National Strength and Conditioning Association. In general, these organizations test the trainer for his or her knowledge of physiology and understanding of training principles.

Is a personal trainer for you? That's a question that only you can answer. The vast majority of weight trainers have never employed a personal trainer, instead relying on books or friends.

If you're not one of the majority, the best advice is to shop wisely by interviewing, checking credentials, and asking for references, just as you would if you hired any other service provider.

With your home gym equipped, or a gym membership card in hand, and an eager training partner lined up, you're ready to start your training. Let's move on.

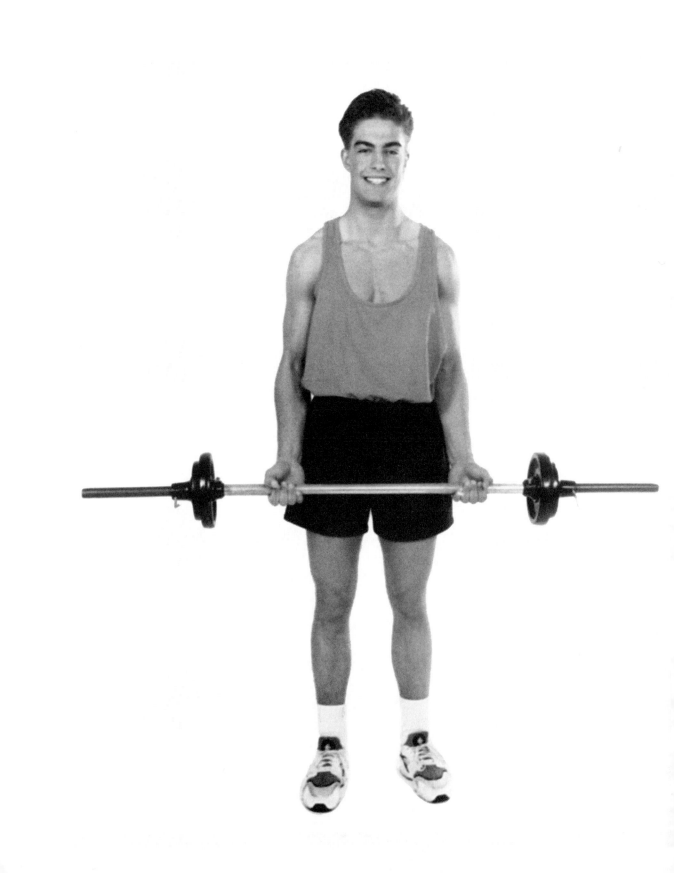

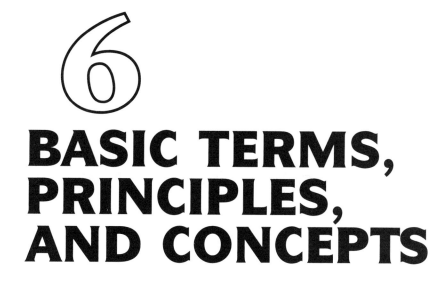

BASIC TERMS, PRINCIPLES, AND CONCEPTS

A road sign on a highway. A culinary term in a recipe. A parts list to assemble a Christmas toy. All are guides that enable the driver, cook, or assembler to successfully negotiate the respective task.

An understanding of the basic "language" of any activity increases the likelihood that the activity will be correctly performed. That premise holds true for weight training.

The remainder of this chapter will develop a common language and collection of concepts that we can rely on for clarity of communication throughout the remainder of the book. Let's begin with the term that has drawn you to this book—*weight training.*

BASIC TERMS

Weight Training

Weight training is exercise that adds resistance to any one of the body's natural movements. The resistance is added to make the movement more difficult.

Weight training is synonymous with *resistance training.* Weight training became the popular term because "weights"—barbells and dumbbells—were the early devices of weight training. Today, barbells, dumbbells, and weight machines are still the primary stuff of resistance training. But lifting cows, pushing automobiles, or performing pushups and pullups against the resistance of body weight also qualifies as weight training. The defining characteristic is that of *adding resistance to a natural movement.*

The focus of this book reflects the common perception of weight training, where resistance is supplied by barbells and dumbbells.

Repetitions

A repetition, or rep, is one complete exercise movement. One pushup, one curl, and one squat are examples of one rep.

If you're shooting free throws, each free-throw attempt is a rep. Weight-training reps are analogous to counting free throws.

Sets

In weight training, sets are groups of repetitions. The size of the set might be any number of reps, but in this book, most of the sets will be 10 or 15 reps. Whatever the quantity of the group, the concept is the same: A set is a group of reps.

REST PERIOD BETWEEN SETS

How long should you rest between sets? You will probably need to rest two to four minutes between sets. The length of the rest period shortens as conditioning improves the muscles' ability to accommodate training stress.

There are no absolutes about rest periods. Two to four minutes is not mandatory. Your personal level of conditioning determines the length of rest required between sets.

BASIC TRAINING PRINCIPLES

Principles are comprehensive or fundamental laws, the foundation upon which an endeavor or discipline is built. There are principles of economics, principles of biology, and principles of human behavior, and, of course, principles of weight training.

Five principles are the foundation for all successful weight-training programs. All the exercises that follow respect the same five principles. Bigger and stronger muscles result from respecting the five principles.

Principle 1. Resistance Movements: Weight training involves adding resistance to a natural body movement

Raise your hand above your head as if reaching for something on a high shelf. That's a natural movement.

Now raise your hand above your head while holding a rock, bag of sugar, or computer terminal. You've added resistance.

Lifting a hand above the head, squatting, and curling the hand toward the shoulder are all examples of natural movements that you've performed your entire life. They're also three of the primary movements of a weight-training program.

APPLYING THE PRINCIPLE

"Where do I start" is the first question for any new weight trainer. The only way to find out is through experimentation.

Your first several workouts should be spent finding a rough estimate of an appropriate overload weight for all your exercises. Begin the experimentation with a *very* light weight.

Gradually add plates until you arrive at the proper poundage for the 10-repetition overload set (see "Overload," below).

Why spend several workouts to find an appropriate overload weight? There's no need to rush to use maximum weights. Too heavy a weight in the beginning often compromises correct form that can add to the potential for injury. Hence, the workouts spent selecting proper poundages are workouts well spent. Remember, the goals of your weight-training program are long-range.

Start your weight-training program on a solid foundation by following these safety guidelines and practicing correct form.

Principle 2. Overload: The weight-training program must overload the muscles

Muscles that propel your body's movements become stronger and bigger in response to the resistance they are required to work against.

Overloading the muscle—applying resistance close to the muscle's capacity—will make it stronger and bigger. A muscle working near capacity goes through a complex sequence of metabolic processes designed to prepare it for greater capacity the next time it's called into action. The end result is a bigger and stronger muscle.

You're overloading the muscle when you perform an exercise for a maximum number of repetitions with a given resistance. For example, if you can perform 10 repetitions in the squat with 100 pounds on your shoulders, and the tenth rep exhausts your physical capacity, you have effectively overloaded the muscles involved in the squat.

Why is overloading the muscles so important? It's the only way to induce the muscle to strengthen, grow, and change shape. Conversely, if training demands on the muscle are less than overload, the muscles will shrink and weaken, just as surely as the muscles in your arm would atrophy if immobilized in a cast for several weeks.

APPLYING THE PRINCIPLE

The first set of each exercise, which doesn't count as an overload set, is a movement-specific warm-up. Most weight trainers have learned that a warm-up improves performance during the actual overload sets. During the warm-up, as the muscles' temperature rises:

- muscles contract with more force;
- tendons and ligaments become more pliable; and
- nerves conduct impulses to and from the muscles faster.

Following the warm-up set, subsequent sets (overload sets) are the real muscle builders. Consisting of 8 to 10 repetitions, these sets are performed with an appropriately heavier weight as discussed above. These sets place greater demands on the muscles, forcing them to adapt with improved strength and size.

The number of overload sets range from one to five, depending on your experience, age, and objectives.

Beginners
- One warm-up set of 15 repetitions.
- Two overload sets of 8 to 10 repetitions.

Advanced
- One warm-up set of 15 repetitions.
- Three to five overload sets of 8 to 10 repetitions.

Principle 3. Progressive resistance: As the muscles increase in strength, resistance must be increased

In practice, progressive resistance training means adding weight to the barbell or dumbbell when you're able to do so. It requires mental drive to always try to lift the next-heaviest weight. It takes a lot of effort, but that separates the gainers and no-gainers in a weight-training program.

When do you progress, adding weight to a barbell or dumbbell? The rule of thumb: when you're able to complete ten repetitions with a given weight, increase that weight 10 percent for your next workout. The increased weight will reduce your repetitions during subsequent workouts, perhaps to 8 reps, but that's to be expected.

Once you're able to perform 10 reps with this new, heavier weight, the cycle repeats itself. Again, increase the weight another 10 percent for subsequent workouts.

Progressive resistance training progressively increases your ability to perform. That improved performance is the weight trainer's measure of success.

APPLYING THE PRINCIPLE

When you are able to perform an eleventh rep during your overload set, it's time to add weight to the barbell or dumbbell during your next workout.

As outlined above, choose a new weight that exhausts your ability at 8 to 10 repetitions. A small increase in poundage is usually all that's necessary: perhaps a five- or ten-pound increase in the weight of the barbell (half that much if the exercise calls for dumbbells). Make sure the new weight can be lifted at least eight times during the overload set.

Use this newly selected weight until you once again exceed the 10-rep parameter. Repeat the procedure of increasing the weight.

Principle 4. A combination of strength gains and muscle growth comes most quickly through sets of 8 to 10 repetitions.

I recommend sets of 8 to 10 repetitions. That rep pattern best stimulates the combination of strength gains and muscle growth.

Lower reps (sets of 2 to 6) work best for strength development: There is an argument that slightly more reps (12 reps) work best for short-term bodybuilding rewards, but sets of 8 to 10 reps work best for long-term muscle growth. Remember, if you're a beginner, think long-term.

Principle 5. Rest Between Workouts: The muscles need time between training sessions to recuperate and grow

Muscles need time between training sessions to replenish energy reserves and mend or build tissue.

Overtraining—training before the muscle has had adequate rest—can have serious side effects. To protect against overtraining, most serious bodybuilders rest at least one day between workouts exercising the same body parts. That's why the common three-days-a-week training pattern emerged: One day of training is followed by one day of rest and recuperation.

If muscles aren't given enough posttraining rest, they will lose rather than gain strength. They are also more susceptible to injury.

The above principles are the foundation of all successful weight-training programs. Follow them and you're on the right path to reaching your goals.

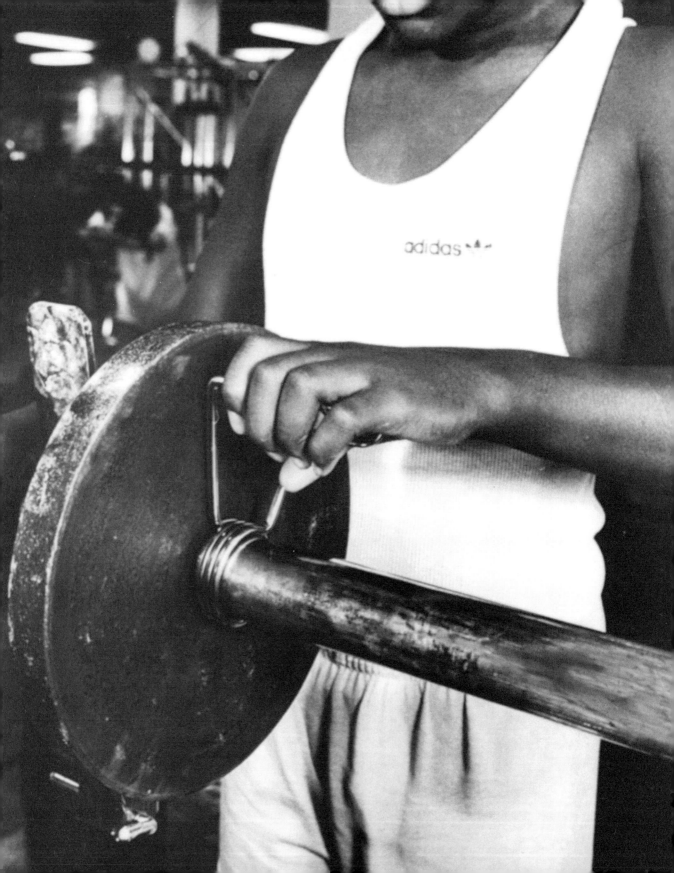

7
BASIC SAFETY RULES

I love taking aerobic-dance classes. The rhythmic music and a high-energy instructor makes the hour of cardiovascular exercise a breeze. But I hated what it did to me—more correctly, what my enthusiasm and stupidity caused me—the day after my very first class.

I could hardly sit without pain. Once sitting, I couldn't stand without pain. Everything hurt. It hurt my pride as well when my wife told me that I should have listened to my own advice: Every new physical activity should be initiated with moderation. I knew not to start a running program by sprinting up a hill, or a weight-training program by lifting as much as I could, and take my word, I know to never again start an aerobics program by kicking as high as I possibly can.

Some "injuries," like minor soreness, can be expected anytime you begin a new physical activity. Not every injury can be avoided, any more than every forest fire can be prevented, but there are ways of preventing serious injuries.

SUPERVISION

Imagine the danger inherent in learning to drive without a supervisor. Sure, Mom or Dad gave you an ear-banging every time you burned the clutch or scraped the curb, but it could have been a lot worse without them sitting beside you, pecking away.

Having an experienced supervisor along for the ride makes weight training less dangerous too. While weight training, with or without a supervisor, ranks well down the list of injury-producing athletic activities, supervision increases the odds that you'll enjoy accident-free weight-training experience.

Personal supervision is particularly valuable when trying an exercise for the first time. Sure, somewhere there are pictures and text that describe all four thousand exercises ever tried in a weight room, and most gyms are lined with mirrors for personal feedback. Nothing, however, replaces the on-the-spot critique of a knowledgeable supervisor. He or she can recognize potential problem situations before they end in injury.

This book is a surrogate supervisor, directing you in the correct technique to perform an exercise. Frankly, it would benefit you to have personal supervision every time you lift weights, but in lieu of that, this book offers the next-best option. Carefully read the instructions. And follow the instructions. Don't improvise. When in doubt, stop. Ask for advice from an experienced friend. As a last resort, send me a personal note in care of the publisher.

WARM-UP

Before Whitney Houston walks on stage for a concert, she warms her vocal cords in her dressing room. It behooves the weight trainer to follow suit.

A warm-up actually raises the temperature of the muscles. Just like Whitney's vocal cords, warm weight-training muscles have greater capacity for strength and endurance.

The warm-up also reduces injuries by increasing the amount of synovial fluid in the joint and routing more blood to the specific muscles involved in the exercise. As mentioned earlier in the book, the warm-up prepares muscles and connective tissue (tendons and ligaments) for the training stresses.

The best advice for warm-ups prior to weight training?

1. Five to ten minutes of aerobic activity—exercise bike, rowing machine, or calisthentics involving the whole body—before that first set of a weight-training exercise.
2. For each weight-training exercise, do a first set of 15 repetitions. That high-rep first set warms the specific muscles involved with the exercise movement.

Don't neglect the warm-up. That measly ten-minute investment returns superior performance while reducing the potential for injury.

- **Warm-up Before, Stretch After**

There is some confusion between stretching and warm-up. They are not the same thing, nor should they be done at the same time.

The warm-up, described above, is performed as a prelude to intense training. The warm-up allows the muscles to gradually elongate to the point appropriate for the weight-training exercise. That's the reason for the 15-rep warm-up set.

After exercising is the most effective and safest time to stretch. Experts believe that when your muscles are warm and pliable, you are less likely to injure yourself from stretching.

Don't confuse warming up with stretching. If you replace stretching for your warm-up, you could increase the potential to tear your cold, inflexible muscles.

This in no way is meant as advice to avoid stretching. There are benefits. Read on.

- **Stretching Improves Strength**

Health magazine reports that a recent study by a University of New England biomechanist, Gregory Wilson, suggests that routine stretching and limbering of shoulder and chest muscles increases strength during the bench press.

Lifters who did limbering stretches improved their bench presses by 5.5 percent (5 to 25 pounds, depending on the beginning strength of each lifter) over the two-month study. The control group that didn't stretch showed no strength gains.

Wilson explains that a muscle is like a rubber band, and stretching a muscle will help extend its reach while allowing it to snap back with greater force.

CHECK THE EQUIPMENT AND THE AREA

The following safety suggestions focus on the free-weight equipment that is described and illustrated throughout the book.

- Clear the floor and return weights to their proper storage place.

Neatness can prevent accidents, such as a trip over unattended free weights on the floor.

- Load bars carefully and evenly.
- Tighten plates and check that collars are secure before you lift.
- Be aware of any space limitations that might interfere with proper execution of an exercise.
- Keep an eye open for other people training in the same area. Accidents can be avoided by being aware.

SPOTTERS

The need for spotters has been repeatedly mentioned throughout the book. There are certain exercises that should never be performed without a spotter. Let's address from a safety perspective the exercises that require the attendance of a competent spotter.

- Bench Press: Many serious accidents have resulted from being pinned under a barbell when bench pressing. Imagine being pinned under a heavy bar that's positioned near your throat.
- Squats: This exercise uses a heavy weight draped across the back of your shoulders and neck. It's no time to get stuck in a squatting position without a spotter.

HEAVY OVERHEAD LIFTS

While weight-training injuries are relatively rare, the most common accidents occur when lifting a weight overhead. The injured are usually beginners trying to lift too much weight.

Imagine thrusting a 100-pound sack of concrete above your head and lowering it in a coordinated movement. That's the predicament a beginner finds himself in when attempting to lift a heavy barbell for the first time.

This is not a blanket condemnation of overhead lifts. Exercises involving overhead lifts are essential for a complete workout, but the lifts must be approached with great caution, especially by beginners.

Beginners should take time, at least several workouts, to gradually find an appropriate training weight for an exercise involving an overhead lift.

Don't end a workout with an unpleasant bump on the head. Take time to perfect technique and find an appropriate weight.

LOADING AND UNLOADING

The second most common cause of weight-training accidents involves loading and unloading a barbell that is sitting atop a bench press or squat stand.

Don't allow an extreme load imbalance to occur while loading or unloading a barbell. For example, if the goal is to have three 25-pound plates on each end of a bar, alternate the loading of the plates from end to end. Placing three 25s on one end before placing a single plate on the opposite end will cause the bar to fall.

Alternately load the plates, securely tightening the collars when finished loading. Follow the same process when unloading the weights.

PROTECT OLD INJURIES

Before weight training, make an injury inventory. An old injury is often a more likely candidate for injury than a never-before-injured muscle, tendon, or bone.

Protecting that old injury might require nothing more than special consideration in exercise selection. Given two exercises working the same muscle group, a bad knee, elbow, or ankle might be able to endure the stress of one exercise but not the other.

The old injury might require a protective elastic bandage, brace, or taping. If an old injury is substantial, it's always best to check with a doctor before embarking on a weight-training program.

DON'T TRAIN TOO MUCH

More is not always better. *Overtraining,* training before the muscle has fully recuperated from a previous training session, precipitates many preventable injuries.

A basic principle of weight training is that muscles need rest from the stress of weight training in order to recuperate for another round of stress. I noted this earlier in the book in regard to foundations of a successful training program. The focus here is preventing injuries.

Microscopic damage to tissue that results from intense training must be repaired through the body's natural recuperative process. That takes time and rest.

The best advice is to respect the recommended sequence of rest days between training sessions: Rest at least one day between training sessions, more if soreness is present. Soreness is an indication of minor tissue damage. Wait until the soreness has subsided before again overloading the affected muscles and joints. You can and should exercise if the problem is only minor soreness. But don't overload the muscle; engage in light exercise, which enhances the body's healing powers by increasing circulation in the sore muscles.

RETURNING AFTER A LAYOFF

Approach training with caution following an extended layoff. Remember that your muscles are no longer conditioned for an intense overload.

The best advice is to spend several workouts training with moderately heavy weights, a weight in which 10 reps are *easy* rather than an overload. You might be able to perform 12 to 14 reps with such a weight, but that's all right. It's better to spend several workouts reacclimating to training stress, rather than several subpar workouts as a result of extremely sore muscles.

Resuming training at your prelayoff intensity is sure to cause extreme soreness and raise the potential for injury. Take time. This is one time when long-range rewards are reached with less rather than more effort.

With basic safety rules in mind, you're ready to begin your training program. Read on.

PART

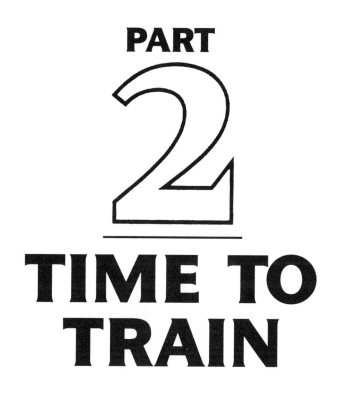

2

TIME TO TRAIN

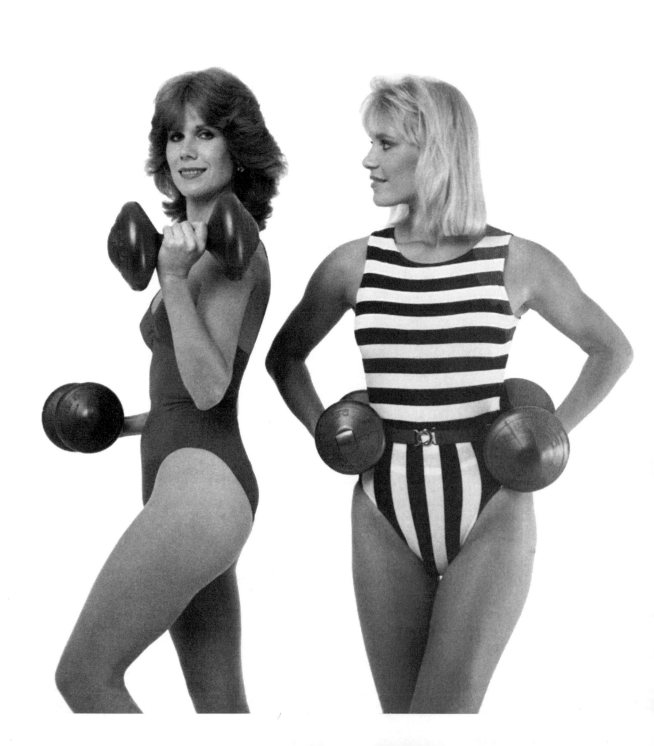

8

TIME TO TRAIN: THE BASIC WORKOUT

If you've read the previous seven chapters, you're ready for a manageable workout. You can accomplish the following eight exercises with a set of adjustable-weight dumbbells, a barbell, a bench, and a block of wood.

After several weeks of the Basic Workout to put you in a training groove, you can add exercises to meet your specific training goals. But now's the time for a full-body workout that will build a foundation for further training.

TRAINING GOAL
Complete eight exercises during each workout that work all major muscle groups: legs, hips, chest, back, shoulders, arms, and abdominals.

GENERAL WARM-UP
Begin the workout with five to ten minutes of general calisthentics or aerobic exercises to prepare all of your five hundred muscles for a cooperative, coordinated effort.

SETS AND REPS
   Warm-up Set. Each exercise begins with one set of 15 reps as a movement-specific warm-up. That means a set with a super-light weight just to get your muscles ready for the more intense work ahead.

What's the right weight? That depends on your level of strength. You can find your level only through trial and error. As a rule of thumb, start light. You've got many workouts to find your exact weight.

Work Sets. Following the warm-up set, perform two to five sets of 8 to 10 repetitions per exercise. Beginners start with two work sets per exercise. What's the right weight for the work set? Again, it's a matter of trial and error. It's going to be heavier than the weight used for the warm-up set, but it will probably take you several workouts to figure out what weight to use. The weight will also vary depending on the specific exercise and body part. The number of sets will increase consistent with your improving physical capacity. You may perform different numbers of sets for different exercises.

DAYS PER WEEK
Begin with two or three workouts per week with at least one day of rest between workout days.

TIME REQUIRED
You will spend twenty to forty minutes per workout, depending on the number of sets per exercise and the training sequence that you choose. (See "Training Sequence," below.)

TRAINING SEQUENCE
The best sequence for most people is to start with the more massive muscle groups, because they require more energy to train. Most people follow up by training the smaller muscle groups. That means a training sequence like the following:

Thighs and Hips→Chest→Back→Shoulders
→Biceps→Triceps→Forearms→
Abdominals

You can complete the above-suggested training sequence by choosing between two equally effective options.

Option 1. Complete all sets of a given exercise(s) that affect any one body part before training the next body part. That is, finish training your thighs and hips before training your chest.

Option 2. *Circuit Train.* Do one set for one body part, then immediately move to an exercise for another body part. One set per body part—thighs and hips through abs—is one complete circuit.

Circuit training shortens workout time by eliminating rest periods between sets.

EXERCISE DESCRIPTIONS OF THE BASIC WORKOUT

Whichever option you choose, it's time to train. Pay close attention to the exercise directions that follow. In fact, keep the book open while you train.

THIGHS AND HIPS

Lunge

FOCUS: BUTTOCKS AND THIGHS (FRONT, REAR, INSIDE)
SECONDARY EMPHASIS: LOWER BACK, CALVES

Beginner's Note   Practice the technique without weights for the first several workouts before adding resistance. Once you're able to perfectly execute 15 repetitions with your body weight, add appropriately weighted dumbbells. And be sure to make the transition to dumbbells rather than barbells. Dumbbells are easier to balance and are just as effective.

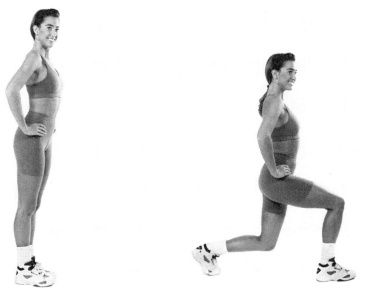

CORRECT TECHNIQUE

Starting Position   Stand upright with feet placed shoulder-width apart, hands on hips or at your sides as counterbalances.

1. Keeping head up and back straight, take a long step forward with either foot. Plant your foot and drop your hips until the lead thigh is parallel to the floor. Your knee should be bent approximately 90 degrees and your front foot should be flat against the floor.

2. Push backward and upward with the lead foot until you are standing erect at the starting position. Repeat with the opposite leg. That's one rep. Alternate legs until you've completed the required number of repetitions—that's one set.

CHEST

Regular Push-ups

FOCUS: CHEST (PECTORALS)
SECONDARY EMPHASIS: FRONT OF SHOULDERS (FRONT DELTOID)

Beginner's Note This is often a difficult movement for beginners: How many times in your life have you pushed your arms in front of your chest with full force? If you're unable to perform the recommended rep count, start with Bent-Knee Push-ups (see p. 130). The Bent-Knee variety takes less strength to perform.

   If you're too strong for Regular Push-Ups, try Weighted Push-Ups or Push-Ups Off Bench to increase resistance to your movements (see pp. 131–132).

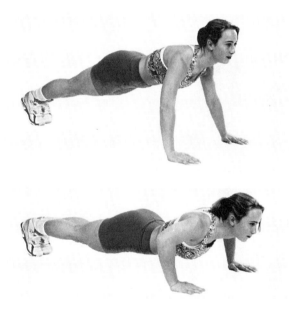

CORRECT TECHNIQUE

Starting Position Extend your arms below your shoulders with your body held rigidly straight. Don't allow your stomach or lower back to sag.

1. Under control throughout the movement, lower your body until your chest gently touches the floor.

2. Press upward to the starting position, keeping your body straight during the movement.

SHOULDERS

Standing Lateral Raise

FOCUS: OUTER AND FRONT DELTOIDS

Beginner's Note   Standing laterals are often awkward for a beginner. It's another motion that isn't part of daily life. That's why it's wise for you to do one of the following:

1. Disregard rep counts and use a *very* light weight for several workouts until you have developed a coordinated movement and can safely perform the exercise with heavier weights.

2. Have an experienced spotter assist you through the exercise movement. The spotter should grip your forearms throughout the entire movement, guiding the path of the arc.

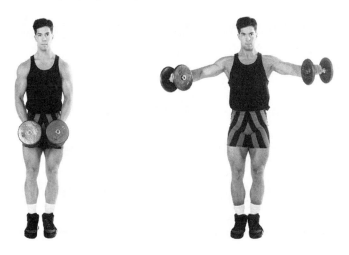

CORRECT TECHNIQUE

Starting Position   Stand with your feet shoulder-width apart, dumbbells hanging at your sides with palms facing your thighs. Your knees can be slightly bent to maintain balance throughout the movement.

1. Raise the dumbbells through a lateral arc to shoulder height. Keep your arms rigid throughout the movement. The backs of your hands should face the ceiling when the dumbells reach shoulder height.

2. Lower the dumbbells by returning through the same lateral arc to the starting position. That's a rep.

• Your elbows may be kept slightly bent, but rigid, throughout the movement. A straight or bent elbow depends on personal taste.

BACK

One-Arm Dumbbell Row

FOCUS: UPPER BACK
SECONDARY EMPHASIS: BICEPS AND REAR DELTOID

Beginner's Note The one-arm dumbbell row was selected for two important reasons: safety and effectiveness. Placing your hand on the bench increases stability, thereby increasing safety, but effectiveness is not compromised. A single dumbbell permits a complete range of motion for the affected muscles.

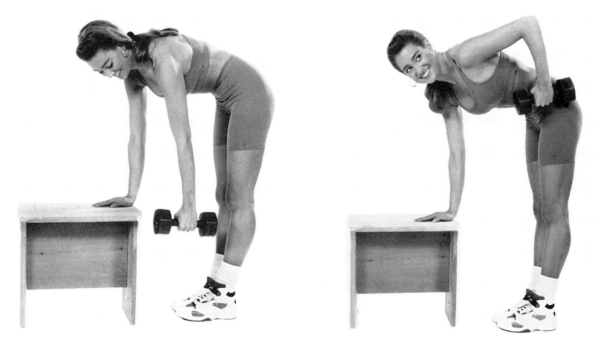

CORRECT TECHNIQUE

Starting Position With your hand on a bench, back straight and parallel with the floor, let the dumbell hang toward the floor.

1. Passing your elbow close to your side, pull the dumbbell upward.

2. Lower the dumbbell toward the floor until you've fully stretched your upper back, shoulder, and arm at the low position. That's a rep.

3. After completing a set with the dumbbell in one hand, switch sides and repeat the exercise on the opposite side.

BICEPS

Seated Dumbbell Biceps Curl

FOCUS: BICEPS
SECONDARY EMPHASIS: FOREARMS

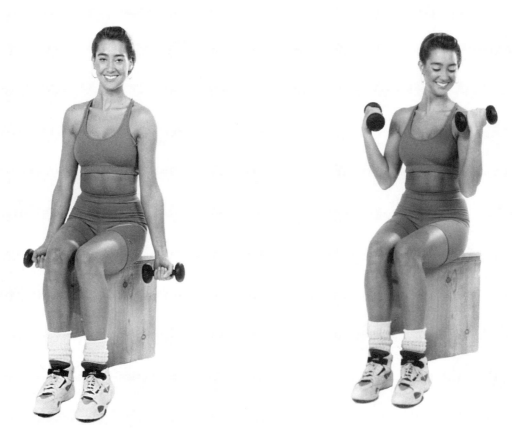

CORRECT TECHNIQUE

Starting Position   Sit on a flat bench. Hang the dumbbells to your sides, palms facing toward the body.

1. Without swinging the dumbbell to enhance acceleration, curl the dumbbells through a semicircle to your chin. Your elbows remain down, your upper arm remains pressed to the body, and your palms rotate upward throughout the movement.

2. Lower the dumbbells through the same arc. Repeat with the opposite arm.

TRICEPS

Standing Tricep Kick-Back

FOCUS: TRICEPS
SECONDARY EMPHASIS: REAR DELTOIDS

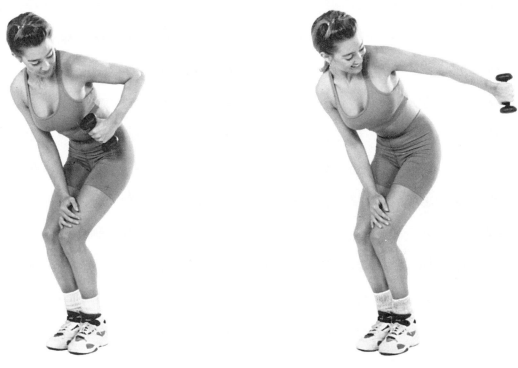

CORRECT TECHNIQUE

Starting Position With knees slightly bent, bend forward at the waist with your upper arm held close to your body and parallel with the floor, a dumbbell hanging down from one hand. Place your free hand on your knee for stability.

1. While keeping your upper arm parallel with the floor, flex your arm until it's straight.

2. Return to the starting position through the same arc, keeping your upper arm parallel to the floor.

• It is important to let your triceps do the work: Don't swing the weight, always lift under control.

FOREARMS

Barbell Wrist Curl

FOCUS: FOREARMS

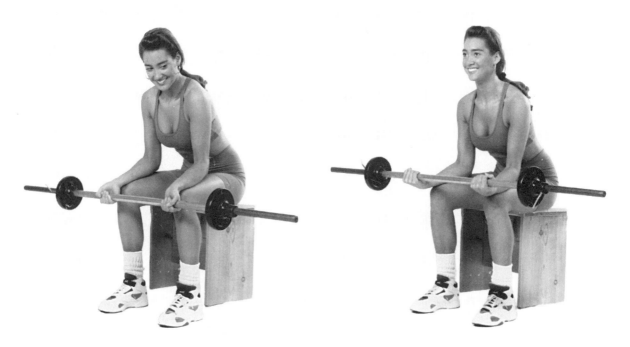

CORRECT TECHNIQUE

Starting Position Sit at the end of the bench, forearms resting on your thighs. Grip the barbell with your palms up. Your wrists should extend beyond your knees.

1. Lower the barbell as low as possible, keeping your forearms pressed against your thighs.

2. Curl the barbell up as high as you can. Be sure to move nothing except the barbell during the lift.

ABDOMEN

Sit-ups

FOCUS: UPPER ABDOMINALS
SECONDARY EMPHASIS: LOWER ABDOMINALS

Beginner's Note   Sit-ups are simple, but there are several precautions to be noted before you begin. Don't pull on your neck with your hands clasped behind your head. If regular sit-ups are too hard for you, place your hands on your stomach—moving the weight of your hands and arms toward your waist will lower the resistance on your abdominals.

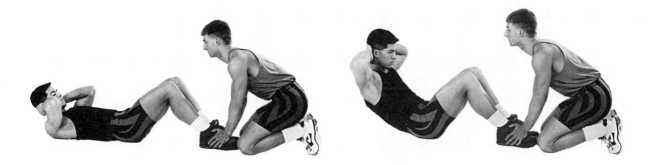

CORRECT TECHNIQUE

Starting Position   Lie on your back with hands clasped behind your neck (holding an appropriately weighted dumbbell if strength permits). Your knees should be bent. Have a training partner hold your feet or slip them into or under a secure restraint.

1. Slowly sit up until your torso is at a 45-degree angle to the floor.

2. Under control, return to the starting position, retaining the bend in your knee throughout the movement. That's a rep.

● Train your abdominals using the same number of sets and reps as with any other muscle group. Continually increase the resistance as your strength allows, using a dumbbell held behind the neck.
● Twisting your torso as you rise is a way of varying the exercise and expanding the range of muscular adaptation.

That's the end of your Basic Workout. What are your options at this point? There are several.

After you've had a few weeks to adjust to the stress of training, you might move on to spot training. You can focus on specific body parts, adding exercises to your Basic Workout.

What if you want to stick with an eight-exercise full-body program but are tired of the same eight exercises? That's easy. Simply replace the eight exercises with eight new ones from the spot-training list. One new exercise from each body-part category makes a whole new full-body routine.

You can also develop a new full-body routine while still focusing on a specific body part. Just choose a new exercise for each body part, then add one or two more for an area of particular concern. In the appendix there is a workout chart to mark your exercises and your progress.

Isn't it wonderful to have so many choices in a weight-training program?

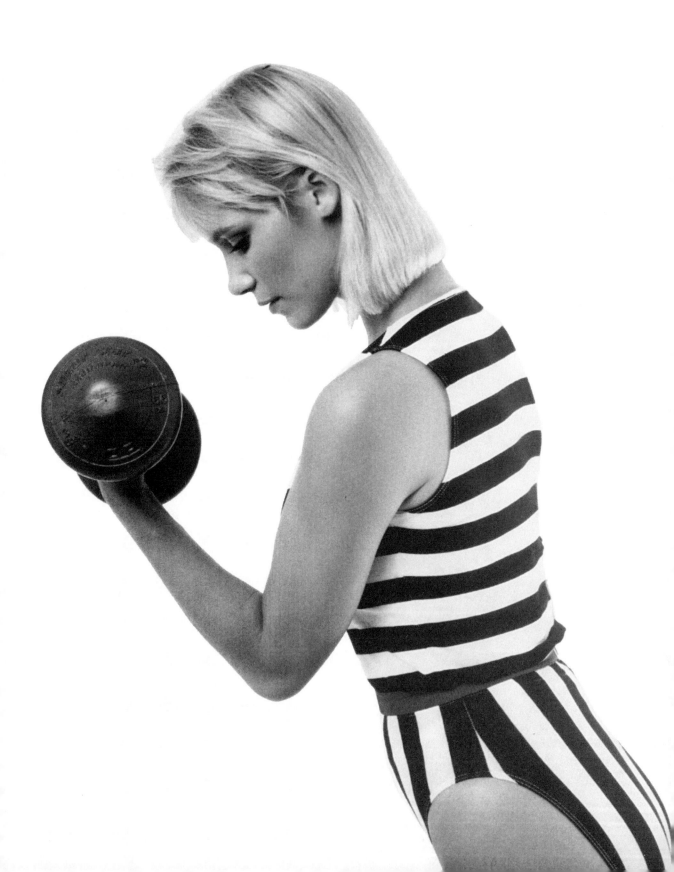

SPOT-TRAINING PROGRAM

Do you want broader shoulders? Firmer hips and thighs? You're in luck. Spot training can transform the size, shape, and tone of shoulders, hips, and thighs—any muscle group. This transformation of a muscle through weight training is called body sculpting. In short, spot training is body sculpting.

You already know that spot *reducing* doesn't work. You can't sweat, jiggle, shake, or wiggle fat away from a particular spot. Sauna wraps, rubber suits, and vibrating belts don't work. Neither does exercise. That's because *fat* is lost uniformly from all parts of the body when you diet or exercise.

Muscles can be selectively trained to change size or shape. That's because weight training, unlike dieting, affects only the muscles being exercised.

Successful spot training requires careful exercise selection. That means choosing the exercises that work the muscles you want to change. Want a firmer derriere? Choose exercises that work the muscles of the derriere. Want shapelier calves? Choose exercises that work the calves.

This chapter will make it easier to choose exercises that meet your specific training goals. The exercises are categorized according to body part and include exercises for the abdomen, back, biceps, calves, chest, forearms, shoulders, thighs and hips, and triceps. Some of these exercises might already be part of your basic routine. Here's what to do.

• Adding Exercises

To emphasize a particular body part, add one or more spot-specific exercises to your basic routine. The number of exercises added depends on your time commitment, condition, and specific goal. Mixing and matching—three added calf exercises and one added chest exercise—might be right for you. A single added biceps exercise might be right for me.

• Sets and Reps

Do one set of 15 reps as a movement-specific warm-up.

Do two to five sets of 8 to 10 repetitions per exercise.

The number of sets is determined by your condition. You may perform different numbers of sets for different exercises.

• Days Per Week

Work out two or three days per week, with at least one day of rest between workouts that focus on the same muscle group.

SPOT TRAINING: ABDOMEN

Sit-ups

FOCUS: UPPER ABDOMINALS

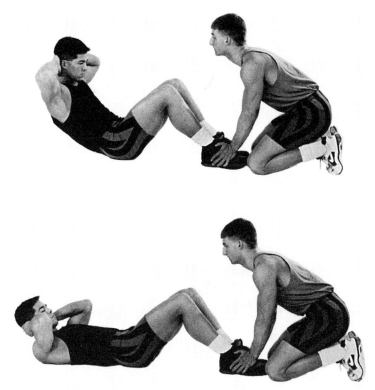

CORRECT TECHNIQUE

Starting Position   Lie on your back with hands clasped behind your neck (holding an appropriately weighted dumbbell if strength permits). Your knees should be bent. Have a training partner hold your feet or slip them into a secure restraint.

1. Slowly sit up until your torso is at a 45-degree angle to the floor.

2. Under control, return to the starting position, retaining the bend in your knee throughout the movement. That's a rep.

  • Train your abdominals using the same number of sets and reps as with any other muscle group. Continually increase the resistance with a dumbbell held behind your neck as your strength allows.

VARIATION: SIT-UP, LEGS ON BENCH

MASTER EXERCISE: SIT-UP

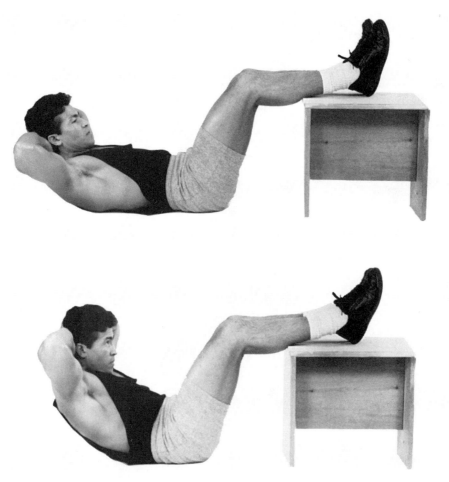

TECHNIQUE VARIATIONS

• Sometimes called a "crunch" sit-up, the angle of your back to the floor ranges from 20 to 40 degrees at the top of the movement.

• Add resistance by placing a dumbbell behind your neck when your strength permits.

Dip Stand Leg Raise

FOCUS: HIP FLEXORS AND LOWER ABDOMINALS

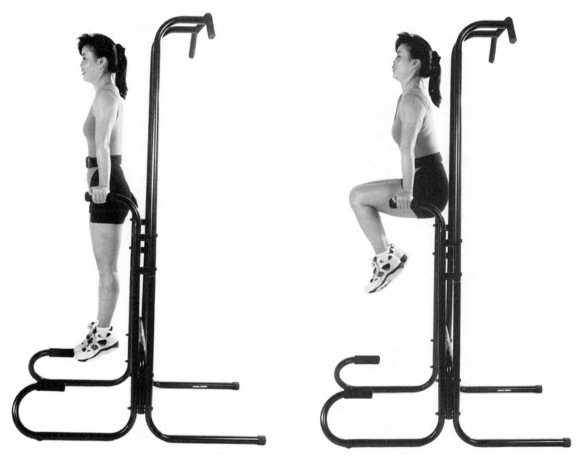

CORRECT TECHNIQUE

Starting Position   Support yourself on the dip bars with straight arms and legs perpendicular to the floor. Maintain a secure grip on the bars.

1. Raise both legs simultaneously, keeping them under control, until your thighs are parallel with the floor.

2. Lower your legs to the starting position. That's a rep.

• For greater resistance, keep your legs straight throughout the movement. When you're able to perform 10 reps with straight legs, add ankle weights to increase the resistance even more.

Leg Tuck

FOCUS: LOWER ABDOMINALS

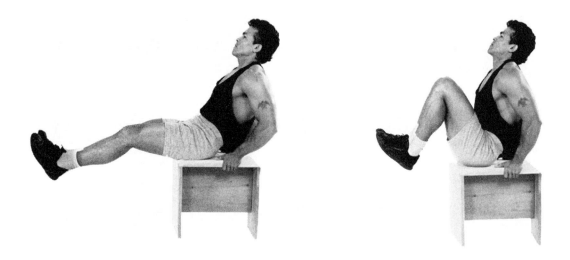

CORRECT TECHNIQUE

Starting Position   Sitting at the end of a flat bench, grip the sides of the bench at a point slightly behind the buttocks. Extend your legs forward while leaning your torso backward.

1. Bend your knees as far toward your torso as possible letting your torso move slightly toward an upright position.

2. Return to the starting position to complete the rep.

Leg Raise on Bench
FOCUS: ABDOMINALS

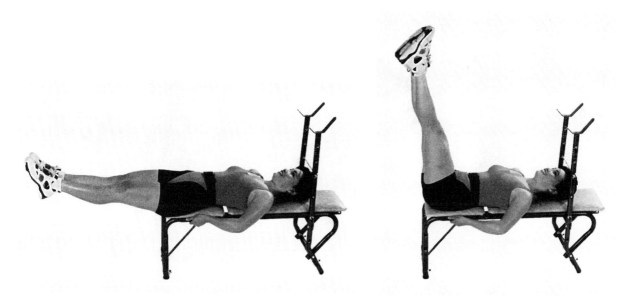

CORRECT TECHNIQUE

Starting Position   Lie on your back, either on the floor or on a bench, with your legs extended in line with your body.

1. Raise both legs simultaneously, keeping them straight and under control, until your feet are above your hips.

2. Lower your legs to the starting position. That's a rep.

- If your current strength is insufficient to perform the exercise with straight legs, bend your legs as necessary.
- Progressively increase resistance by placing an appropriately weighted dumbbell between your feet. *Caution:* Secure the dumbbell with binding to avoid the risk of injury.

Reverse Trunk Twist

FOCUS: ABDOMINALS AND OBLIQUES

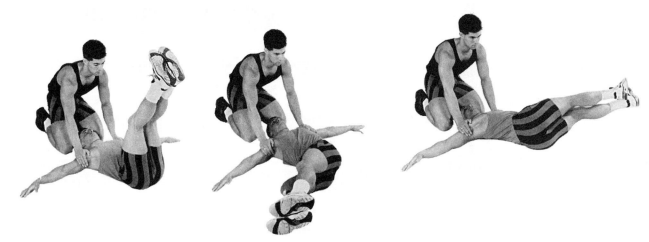

CORRECT TECHNIQUE

Starting Position Lie on your back on the floor, legs vertical to floor, with arms extended to your sides.

1. Slowly lower your knees to one side of your body, keeping your legs perpendicular to your torso throughout the movement.

2. Return to the leg-vertical start position and lower your legs to the opposite side.

3. Return to the start position. That's a rep.

● You can lessen resistance to the movement by bending your knees throughout the exercise. As your ability to perform the exercise improves, the resistance can be increased sequentially by: (1) straightening the legs; and thereafter, (2) adding ankle weights.

SPOT TRAINING: BACK

Good Morning
FOCUS: LOWER BACK (SPINAL ERECTORS)

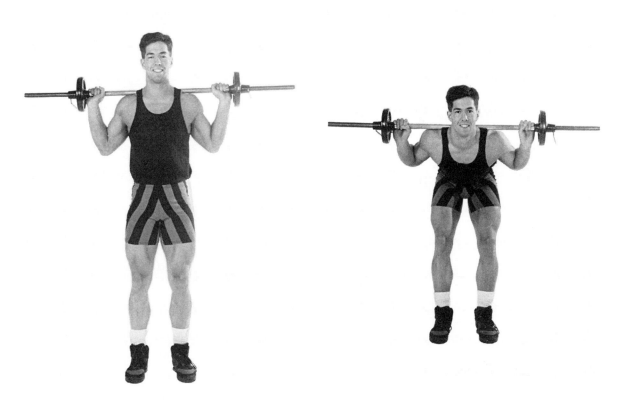

CORRECT TECHNIQUE

Starting Position Stand erect, feet shoulder-width apart, securely gripping a barbell positioned across the back of your neck and shoulders.

1. With back straight and knees slightly bent, slowly bend forward until your torso is parallel with the floor.

2. Ascend through the same arc to the starting position. That's a rep.

Stiff-Legged Barbell Deadlift

FOCUS: SPINAL ERECTORS WITH SECONDARY EMPHASIS
ON THE HAMSTRINGS

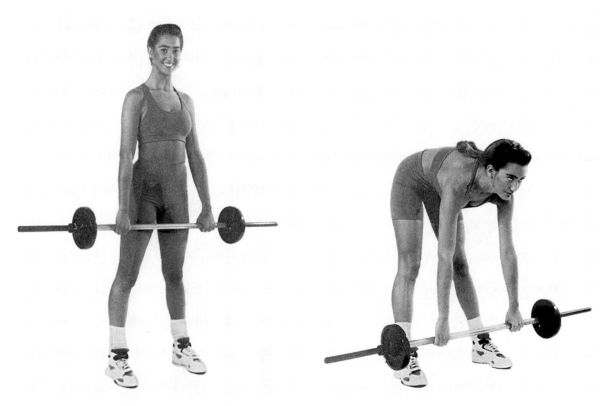

CORRECT TECHNIQUE

Starting Position Stand with your feet parallel and shoulder-width apart, a barbell hanging at arm's length, hands to the outside of your thighs.

1. With knees locked and back kept straight, bend forward at the waist until the barbell plates touch the floor.

2. Ascend through the same arc to the starting position. That's a rep.

• Remain under control thoughout the movement. Don't bounce or jerk the weight off of the floor.

VARIATION: STIFF-LEGGED BARBELL DEADLIFT OFF BLOCK

MASTER EXERCISE: STIFF-LEGGED BARBELL DEADLIFT

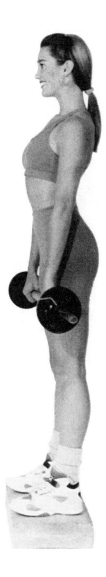
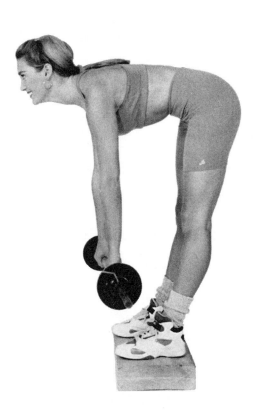

TECHNIQUE VARIATION

• If your flexibility permits, stand atop a low block or other low platform to extend the range of movement several additional inches.

Pull-ups

FOCUS: UPPER BACK

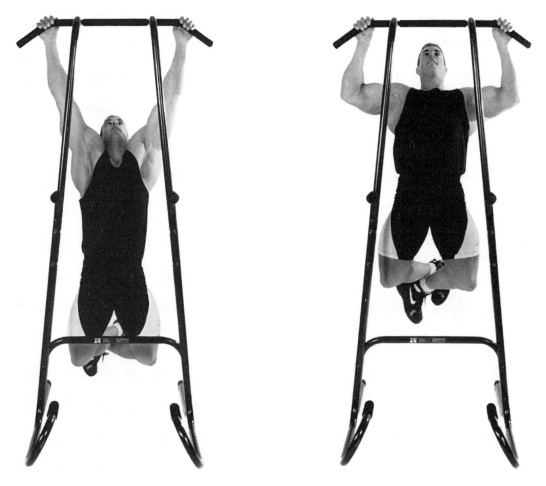

CORRECT TECHNIQUE

Starting Position   Hang from the bar with a secure overhand grip. Hang as low as possible, stretching your lats, arms, and shoulders.

1. Pull your body upward until your elbow is bent less than 90 degrees.

2. Under control, lower your body to the starting position. That's a rep.

   • Vary your grip spacing from workout to workout. The varied grip enhances the range of muscular adaptation.
   • If you're unable to complete a full set, have a spotter assist you.

VARIATION: ASSISTED PULL-UPS

MASTER EXERCISE: PULL-UP

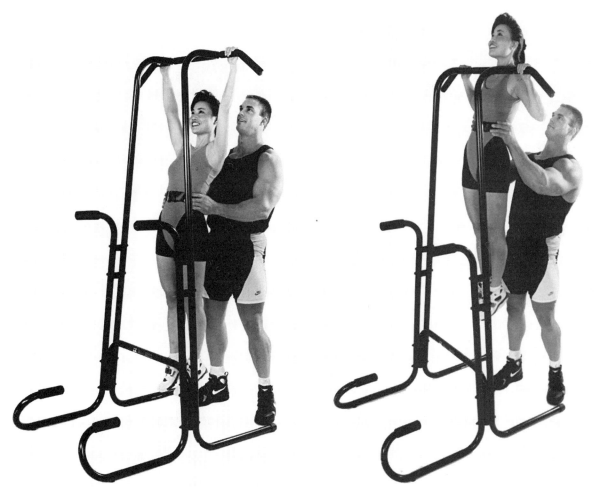

TECHNIQUE VARIATION

• Have a spotter assist by lifting you at your waist or supporting your ankles. The spotter should assist just enough to allow you to complete each rep.

One-Arm Dumbbell Row

FOCUS: UPPER BACK

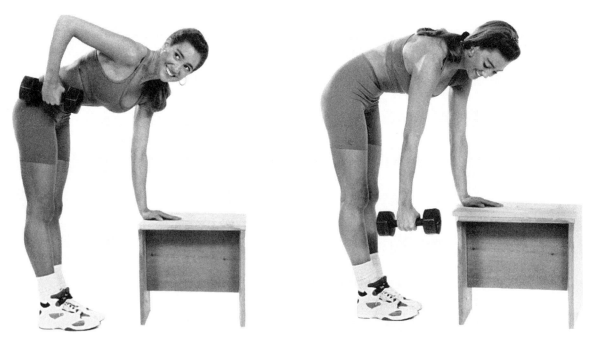

CORRECT TECHNIQUE

Starting Position With your hand on a bench, back straight and parallel with the floor, allow a dumbbell to hang toward the floor.

1. Passing your elbow close to your side, pull the dumbbell upward.

2. Lower the dumbbell toward the floor until fully stretching your upper back, shoulder, and arm at the low position. That's a rep.

3. After completing a set with the dumbbell in one hand, switch sides and repeat the exercise on the opposite side.

Bent-Over Barbell Row

FOCUS: UPPER BACK

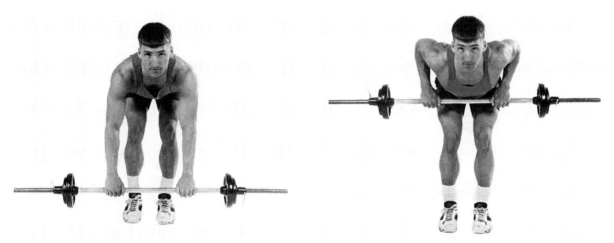

CORRECT TECHNIQUE

Starting Position   Bend at the waist, keeping your back straight and knees slightly bent, and allow a barbell to hang toward the floor.

1. Passing your elbow close to your side, pull the barbell upward until it touches your lower chest.

2. Lower the barbell toward the floor until fully stretching your upper back, shoulder and arm at the low position. That's a rep.

• Don't accelerate the bar with a whiplike motion. Control the movement to protect your lower back.

SPOT TRAINING: BICEPS

Seated Dumbbell Biceps Curl

FOCUS: BICEPS

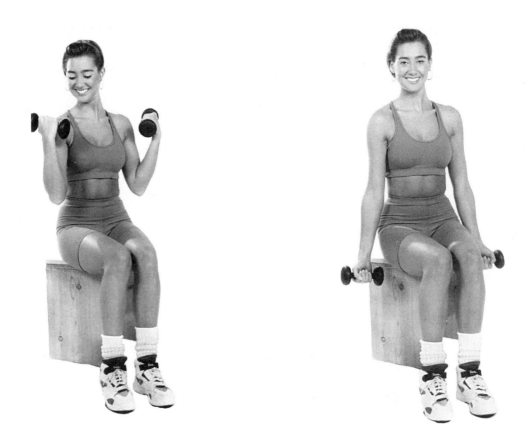

CORRECT TECHNIQUE

Starting Position   Sit on a flat bench. Hang the dumbbells at your sides, palms facing toward the body.

1. Without swinging them to enhance acceleration, curl the dumbbells through a semicircle to your chin. Your elbows remain down, your upper arms are pressed to your body, and your palms rotate upward throughout the movement.

2. Lower the dumbbells through the same arc. Repeat with the opposite arm.

VARIATION: SEATED INCLINE DUMBBELL CURL

MASTER EXERCISE: SEATED DUMBBELL BICEPS CURL

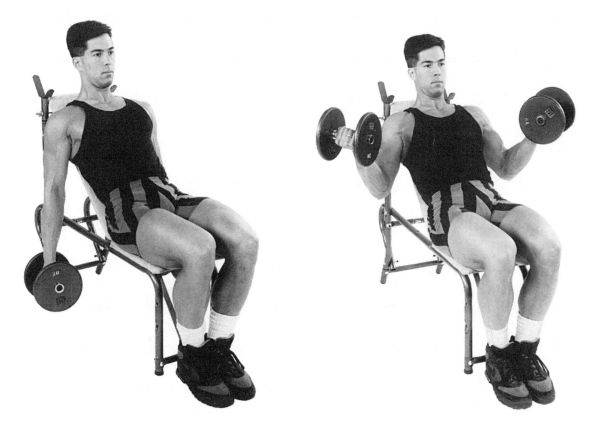

TECHNIQUE VARIATION

• Sit on an incline bench, pressing your back against the backrest positioned at a 45-degree angle. Allow the dumbbells to hang toward the floor.

VARIATION: SEATED ALTERNATE DUMBBELL CURL

MASTER EXERCISE: SEATED DUMBBELL BICEPS CURL

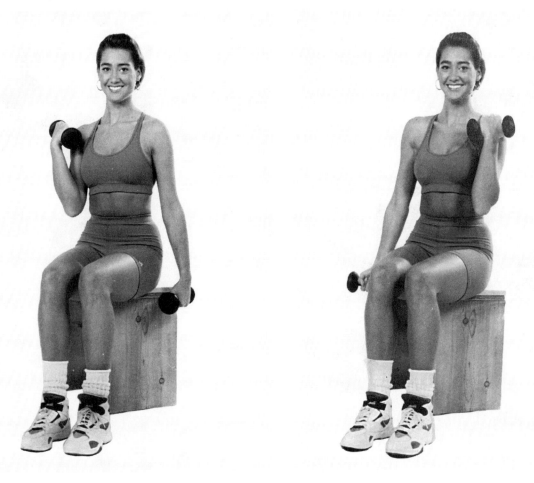

TECHNIQUE VARIATION

• Complete a curl with one arm and immediately follow with the other arm.

VARIATION: STANDING DUMBBELL CURL
MASTER EXERCISE: SEATED DUMBBELL CURL

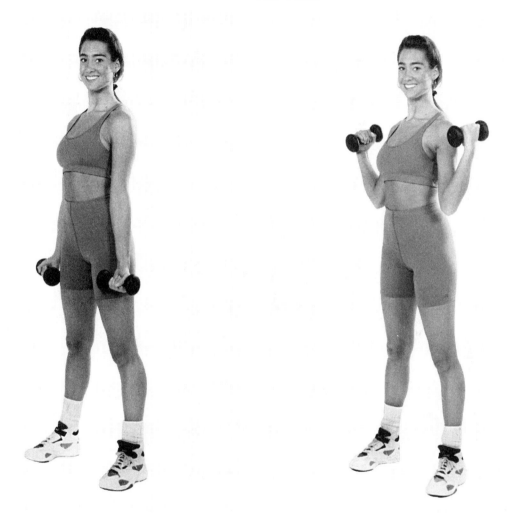

TECHNIQUE VARIATION

• Place feet shoulder-width apart. Take care not to accelerate the dumbbells by leaning forward and swinging your torso at the beginning of the movement.

VARIATION: SEATED CONCENTRATION CURL

MASTER EXERCISE: SEATED DUMBBELL CURL

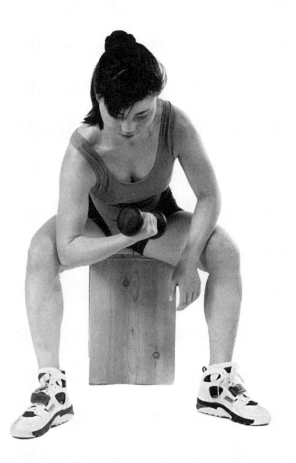

TECHNIQUE VARIATIONS

• Use a single dumbbell, performing a complete set with one arm before exercising the other arm.

• Sit on the end of the bench, positioning the weight between the thighs as pictured. Your upper arm should be braced against the inside of your thigh.

• Concentrate on the biceps as you perform the movement.

Barbell Biceps Curl

FOCUS: BICEPS

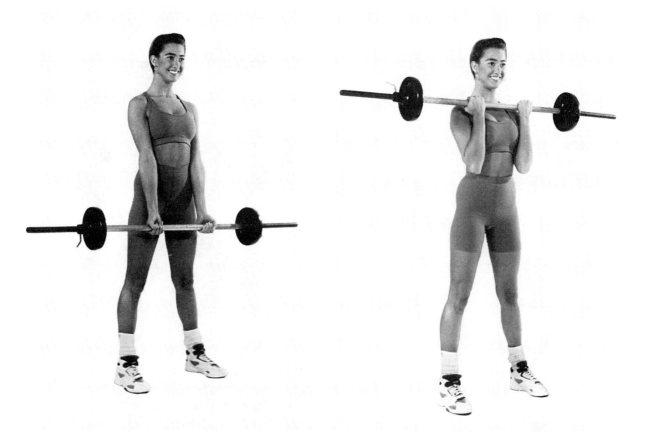

CORRECT TECHNIQUE

Starting Position   Stand erect, feet shoulder-width apart, gripping a hanging barbell with a shoulder-width underhand grip.

1. Maintaining an erect posture, move the bar in a semicircle from the tops of your thighs to a fully flexed elbow position. Use only the strength of your biceps to perform the movement.

2. Return along the same arc to the starting position, retaining control and an erect posture throughout the movement.

   • Try varying the width of your grip from workout to workout. Although all grips work the biceps, varying the grip increases the range of adaptation and makes for a more fully developed muscle.

SPOT TRAINING: CALVES

Seated Toe Raise

FOCUS: CALF

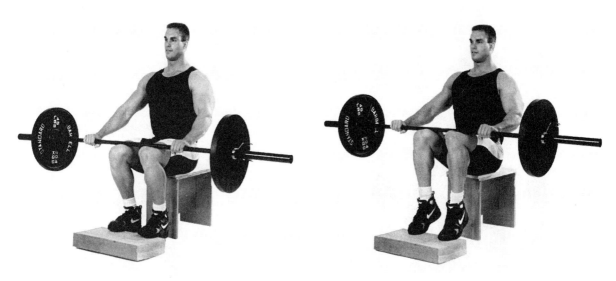

CORRECT TECHNIQUE

Starting Position Sit on the bench with the balls of your feet on a broad block of wood. Position a barbell across your legs, several inches above your knees. Lower your heels as low as possible, stretching your calf muscles in the process. This heels-low, stretched-calf position is the starting point for the exercise.

1. Flex your calves, raising up on your toes as high as possible.

2. Under control, return to the heels-low position. That's a rep.

Standing Single-Leg Toe Raise

FOCUS: CALF

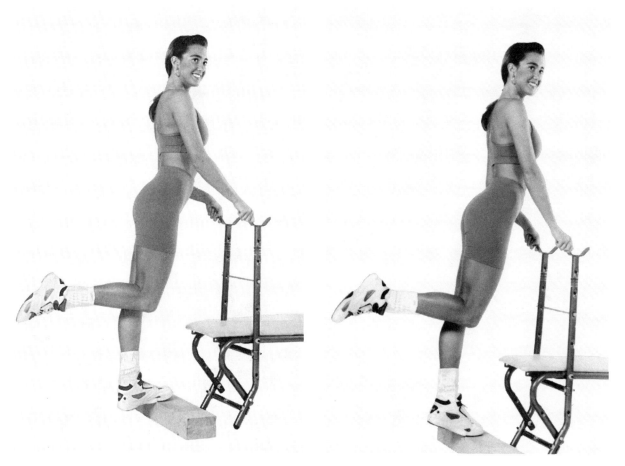

CORRECT TECHNIQUE

Starting Position   Stand erect, eyes forward, the balls of your foot on a broad, stable board approximately 2 inches high. Stabilize your body by holding a bench or bar. Stretch your calf by lowering the heel toward the floor. That's the starting position.

1. Rise up on your toes as high as possible, momentarily holding the contraction of your calf muscle at the top of the movement.

2. Under control, lower your heel to the stretched-calf starting position. That's a rep.

- Weightless single-leg toe raises are excellent for beginners.

VARIATION: SINGLE-LEG TOE RAISE, WEIGHTED

MASTER EXERCISE: STANDING SINGLE-LEG TOE RAISE

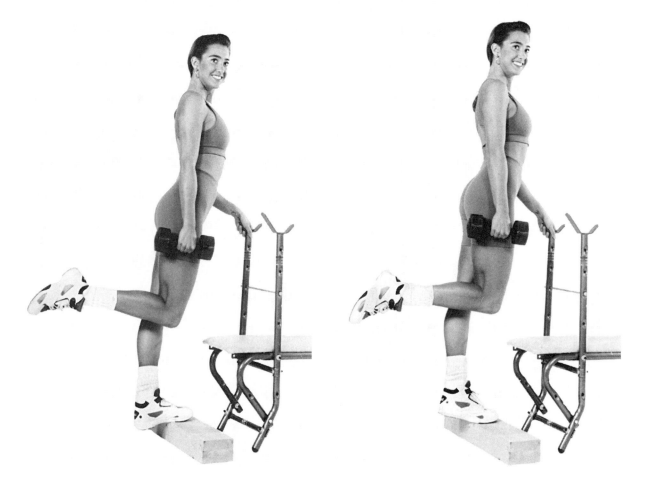

TECHNIQUE VARIATION

• Firmly grip an appropriately weighted dumbbell with one hand, securely gripping a support with the other.

Donkey Toe Raise

FOCUS: CALF

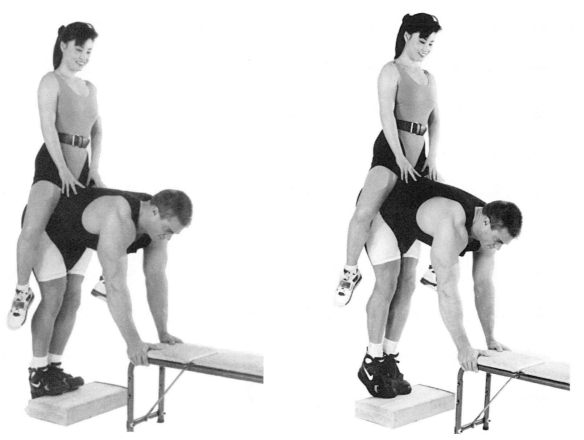

CORRECT TECHNIQUE

Starting Position   Stand with the balls of your feet on a stable board, bending forward at the waist and gripping a bench for stability. Stretch your calf by lowering your heel toward the floor. A training partner carefully and gently positions his/her body atop the hips as pictured. That's the starting position.

1. Rise up on the toes as high as possible, momentarily holding the contraction of your calf muscle at the top of the movement.

2. Under control, lower your heels to the stretched-calf starting position. That's a rep.

• Training partner: Take care in mounting and dismounting your partner. Use a low stool or another bench to reduce the difficulty.

SPOT TRAINING: CHEST

Regular Push-up

FOCUS: PECTORALS

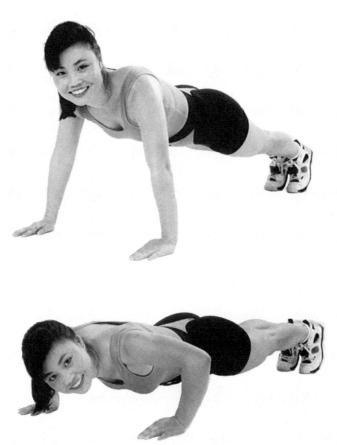

CORRECT TECHNIQUE

Starting Position   Your arms are extended below your shoulders with your body held rigidly straight. Don't allow your stomach or lower back to sag.

1. Under control throughout the movement, lower your body until your chest gently touches the floor.

2. Press upward to the starting position, keeping the body straight during the movement.

VARIATION: DEEP STRETCH PUSH-UP

MASTER EXERCISE: REGULAR PUSH-UP

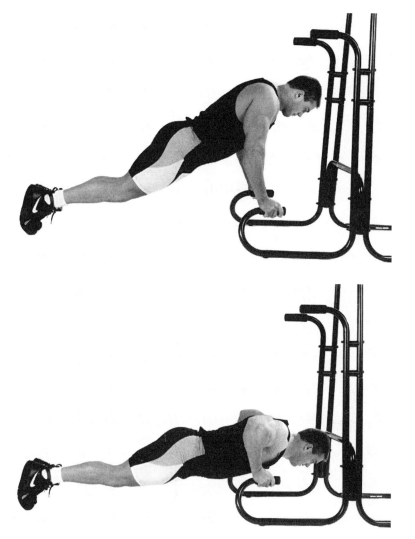

TECHNIQUE VARIATION

• Your hands are elevated on secure blocks or a power stand. The elevation of the hands produces a greater range of motion, effectively increasing the range of muscular adaptation by increasing the range of resistance.

VARIATION: BENT KNEE PUSH-UP

MASTER EXERCISE: REGULAR PUSH-UP

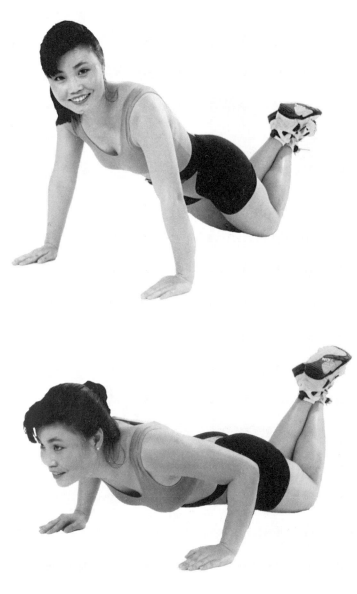

TECHNIQUE VARIATION

• Everything is the same as a regular push-up except that your knees act as support thereby reducing resistance to the movement.

VARIATION: PUSH-UP OFF BENCH

MASTER EXERCISE: REGULAR PUSH-UP

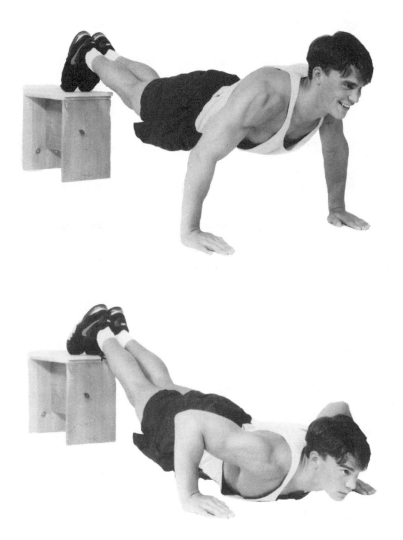

TECHNIQUE VARIATION

• The form is the same as the regular push-up except that your feet are supported above the floor, which will increase resistance to the movement.

VARIATION: WEIGHTED PUSH-UP

MASTER EXERCISE: REGULAR PUSH-UP

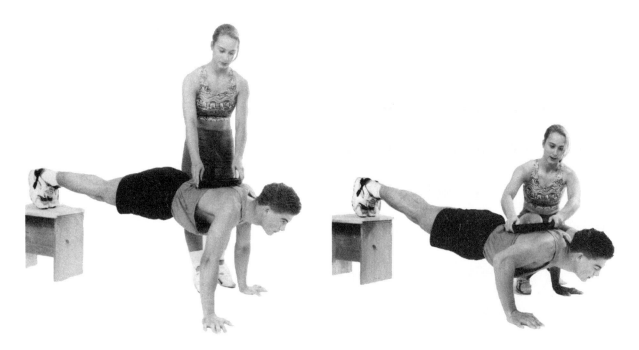

TECHNIQUE VARIATION

• This is similar to the regular push-up except that a training partner secures a barbell plate on your back, increasing resistance to the movement.

Bench Press

FOCUS: CHEST

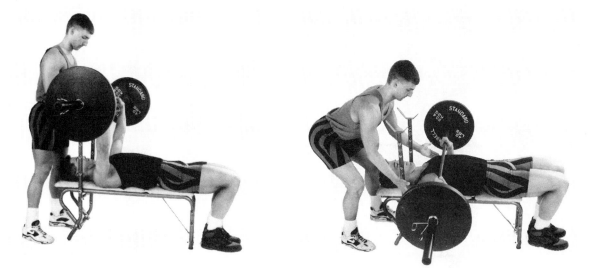

CORRECT TECHNIQUE

Starting Position With your back on the bench, plant your feet firmly on the floor. Grip the bar slightly wider than shoulder-width and support the bar at arm's length. Have a knowledgeable spotter in attendance.

1. Your elbows point out and the bar remains under control as it is lowered to your chest.

2. Return to the starting position by pressing the bar upward, fully extending your arms.

VARIATION: WIDE-GRIP BARBELL BENCH PRESS

MASTER EXERCISE: BARBELL BENCH PRESS

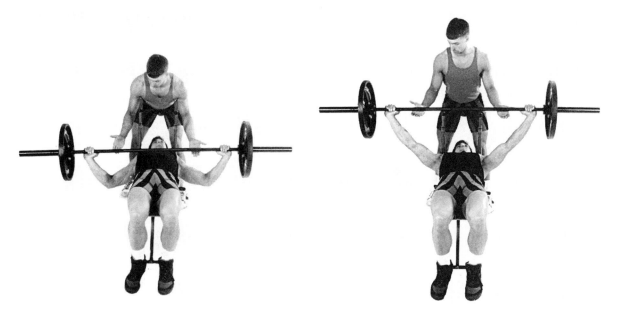

TECHNIQUE VARIATION

• The grip is the only variation in form from the standard barbell press. Grip the bar as wide as possible so long as there is no pain or discomfort in the wrists, hands, elbows, or shoulders.

VARIATION: INCLINE BENCH PRESS

MASTER EXERCISE: BARBELL BENCH PRESS

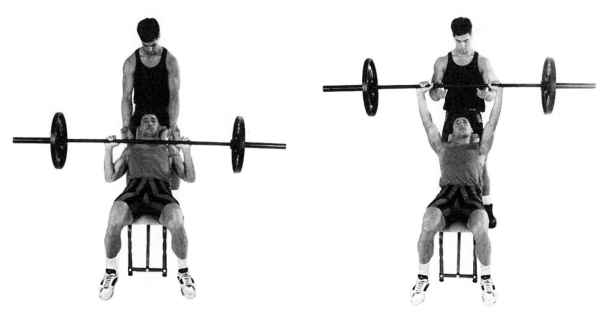

TECHNIQUE VARIATIONS

• The point at which the barbell touches the chest is dependent on the degree of incline. The greater the degree of incline, the closer to the shoulder the bar touches the chest.

• Hand spacing is another important variable. Use multiple hand positions to increase the range of muscular adaptations.

Dumbbell Bench Fly

FOCUS: PECTORALS

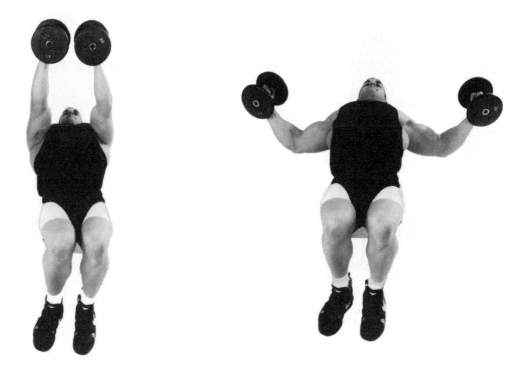

CORRECT TECHNIQUE

Starting Position   Lie on a flat bench, with your feet firmly planted on the floor. Hold the dumbbells at arm's length above the shoulders, palms facing each other and the dumbbells nearly touching.

1. Lower the dumbbells through semicircles until the shoulders and chest are comfortably stretched. Your elbows can bend as much as 45-degrees while lowering the dumbbells. The important point is that tension be focused on your chest.

2. Return the dumbbells to the starting position through the same semicircular path, being careful not to bang the dumbbells at the top. That's a rep.

 • The fly is an "unnatural" movement for beginners, who often lose control of the dumbbells. If you're a beginner, have a knowledge-able spotter assist, or use a *very* light weight for several workouts until you have mastered the form.

VARIATION: DUMBBELL FLY, INCLINE BENCH

MASTER EXERCISE: DUMBBELL FLY

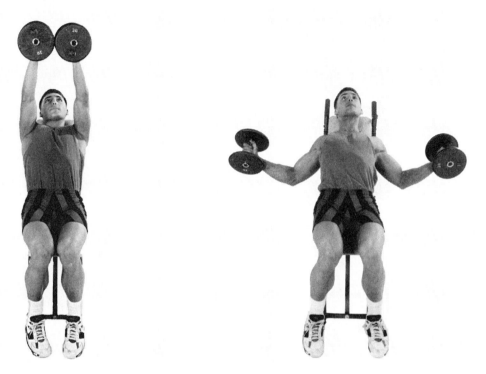

TECHNIQUE VARIATION

- Vary the incline from workout to workout to increase the range of muscular adaptation.

Dip

FOCUS: PECTORALS

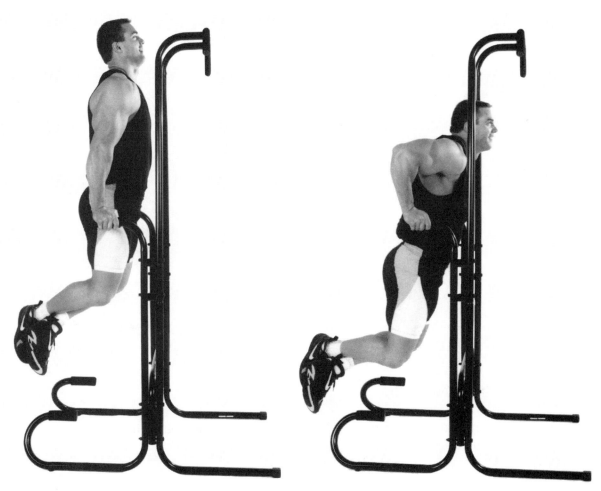

CORRECT TECHNIQUE

Starting Position Support yourself on dip bars, arms straight and shoulder-width apart, body in an erect position, and eyes forward.

1. By bending your elbows, lower your body under control until you feel a comfortable stretch in your shoulder muscles. Your elbows should point in the direction of the bar. Don't bounce at the bottom position.

2. Press yourself upward until you have reached the starting position. That's a rep.

VARIATION: ASSISTED DIP

MASTER EXERCISE: DIP

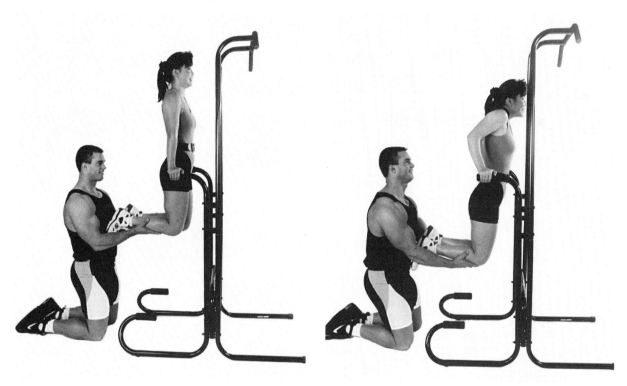

TECHNIQUE VARIATIONS

- Assisted dips allow you to complete a full set of dips if you lack the strength to do them on your own. Have a spotter position his/her hands under your ankles or at your waist and help by applying only as much force as necessary to complete each rep.
- You can also use a bench to partially support your weight if you're training alone.

Bent-Arm Barbell Pullover

FOCUS: UPPER PECTORALS, RIB CAGE

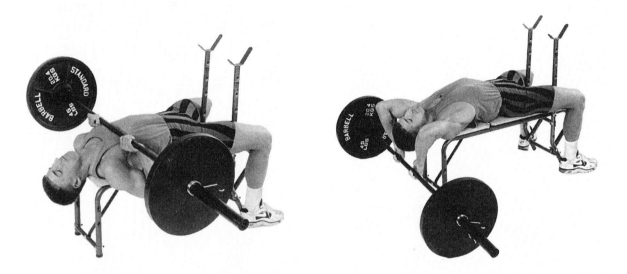

CORRECT TECHNIQUE

Starting Position   Lie on a flat bench with your head extending over one end and your feet on the floor. With a shoulder-width grip, rest an appropriately weighted barbell across your chest. That's the starting position.

1. Keeping your elbows as close to your body as possible, lower the barbell in a semicircular motion from your chest to a fully stretched pain-free position. Your arms remain bent and your back flat against the bench throughout the movement.

2. Return the barbell to your chest through the same arc. That's a rep.

   • Select a bench that permits a full exercise movement without the barbell reaching the floor. Don't bounce or jerk the weight from the floor between reps. Keep your elbows close to your body throughout the movement.

Straight-Arm Barbell Pullover

FOCUS: PECTORALS, RIB CAGE

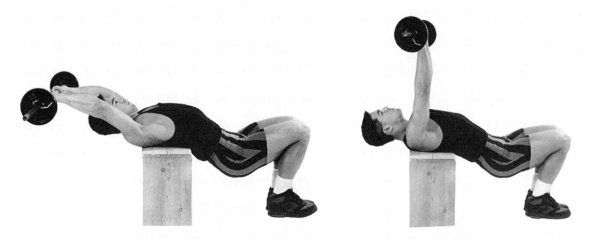

CORRECT TECHNIQUE

Starting Position Lie on a flat bench with your head extending over one end and your feet on the floor. With a shoulder-width grip, extend a barbell arm's length above your chest. That's the starting position.

1. Keeping your elbows forward, lower the barbell in a semicircular motion from your chest to a fully stretched pain-free position. Your arms remain straight and your upper back pressed against the bench throughout the movement.

2. Return the barbell to the starting position through the same arc. That's a rep.

• This exercise can be performed on the floor or across a flat bench. If performed on the floor, don't bounce the weight. In all cases, keep the barbell under control at all times.

VARIATION: STRAIGHT-ARM DUMBBELL PULLOVER

MASTER EXERCISE: STRAIGHT-ARM BARBELL PULLOVER

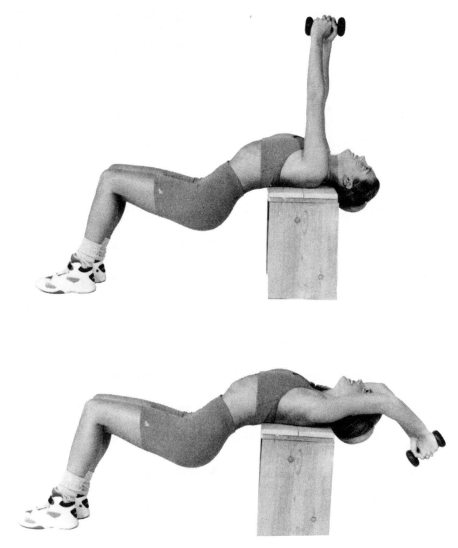

TECHNIQUE VARIATION

• Securely grip a single appropriately weighted dumbbell with both hands. Form is consistent with that described for the master exercise.

Incline Dumbbell Press

FOCUS: UPPER PECTORALS

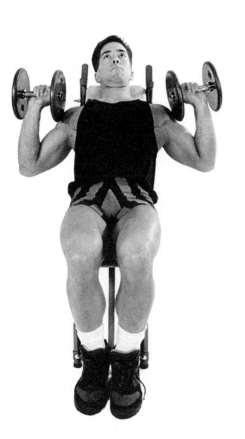
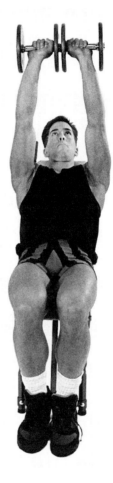

CORRECT TECHNIQUE

Starting Position   Lie back on an inclined bench—20 to 45 degrees—with your feet flat on the floor. Grip dumbbells securely, resting them on your shoulders; palms are facing forward, and elbows are away from your body.

1. Press the dumbbells upward until your arms are fully extended and the dumbbells touch at the top. The important point is to keep tension focused on the chest.

2. Return the dumbbells to the starting position at your shoulders. That's a rep.

SPOT TRAINING: FOREARMS

Barbell Wrist Curl
FOCUS: FOREARMS

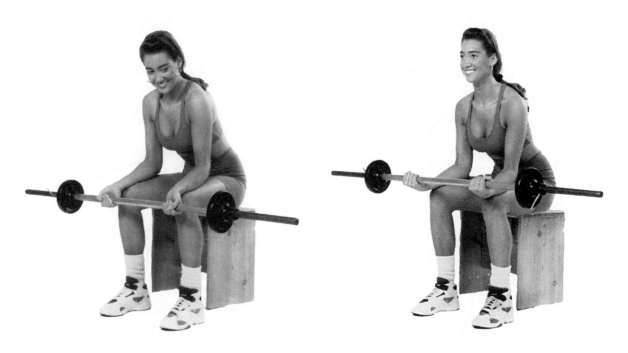

CORRECT TECHNIQUE

Starting Position Sit at the end of the bench, forearms resting on your thighs. Grip the barbell with your palms up. Your wrists extend beyond your knees.

1. Lower the barbell as low as possible, keeping your forearms pressed against your thighs.

2. Curl the barbell up as high as you can. Be sure to move nothing but the barbell during the lift.

VARIATION: REVERSE BARBELL WRIST CURL

MASTER EXERCISE: BARBELL WRIST CURL

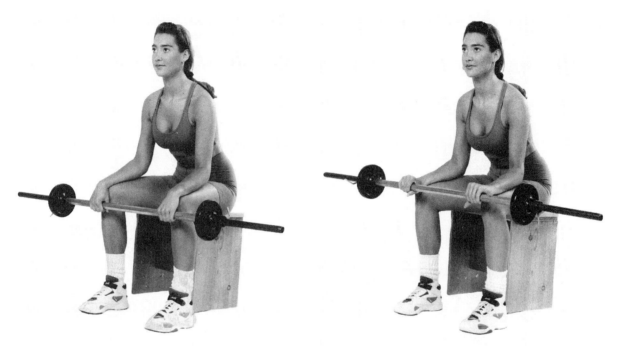

TECHNIQUE VARIATION

- Use an overhead grip for this exercise. All other instructions for the master exercise apply.

VARIATION: DUMBBELL WRIST CURL

MASTER EXERCISE: BARBELL WRIST CURL

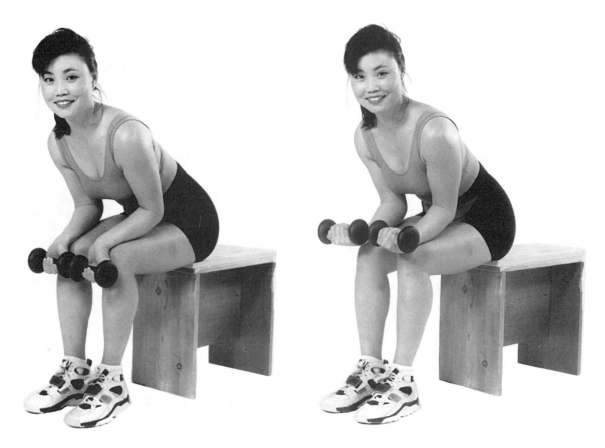

CORRECT TECHNIQUE

• Use dumbells instead of barbell. All other instructions for the master exercise apply.

Hanging Barbell-Behind-the-Back Wrist Curl

FOCUS: FOREARM

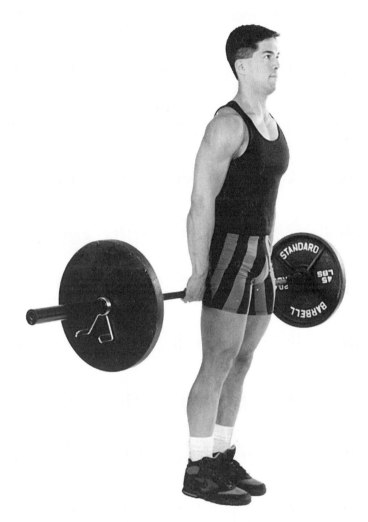

CORRECT TECHNIQUE

Starting Position Stand erect with a barbell hanging behind your back, securely held with an underhand grip (palms away from body).

1. Keeping your arms straight, curl the barbell as high as possible by bending the wrist.

2. Return to the starting position. That's a rep.

SPOT TRAINING: SHOULDERS

Standing Barbell Press
FOCUS: DELTOIDS

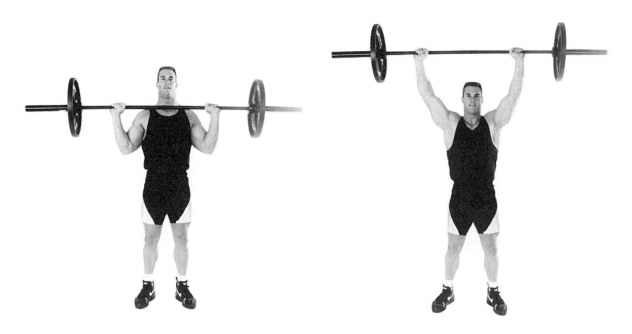

CORRECT TECHNIQUE

Starting Position Position the bar across your shoulders and upper chest with your hands comfortably wider than shoulder-width apart. Feet are parallel and shoulder-width apart, eyes forward.

1. Without arching your back, press the barbell overhead until your arms are fully extended.

2. Pause at the top. Control the barbell as you lower it to the starting position. That's a rep.

- Don't overload the bar at the expense of form.

VARIATION: SEATED BARBELL PRESS

MASTER EXERCISE: STANDING BARBELL PRESS

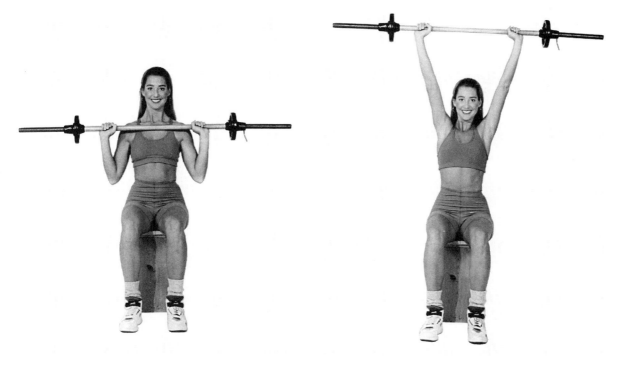

TECHNIQUE VARIATION

• Use the same form as above, but don't allow the lower back to shift while sitting on the bench. Maintain flexed abdominals throughout the exercise movement.

VARIATION: STANDING BEHIND-THE-NECK PRESS

MASTER EXERCISE: STANDING BARBELL PRESS

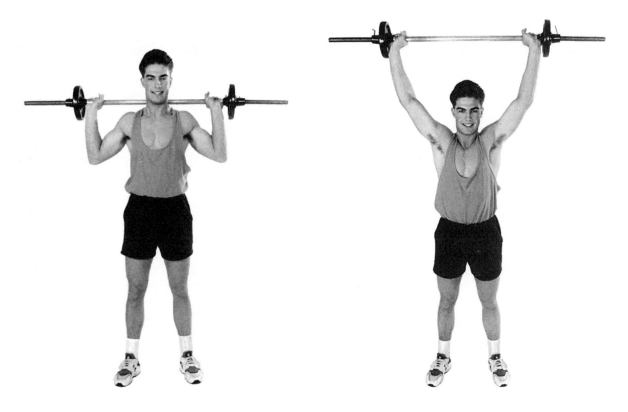

TECHNIQUE VARIATIONS

- The bar is positioned behind the neck, resting on the shoulders.
- Follow the movement pattern as described for the master exercise.

Seated Rear Deltoid Raise

FOCUS: REAR DELTOIDS

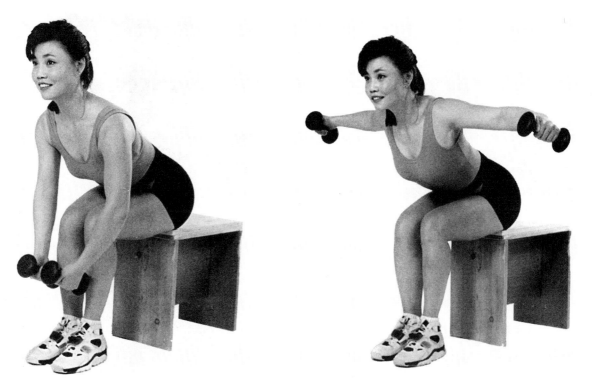

CORRECT TECHNIQUE

Starting Position   Sit at the end of a bench, feet firmly on the floor. Bend forward at the waist and position the dumbbells at arm's length in front of your shins.

1. Keeping your arms rigid (straight or slightly bent) throughout the movement, raise the dumbbells in a semicircular motion until they are parallel to the floor.

2. Lower the dumbbells through the same semicircular path. That's a rep.

Shoulder Shrug

FOCUS: TRAPEZIUS

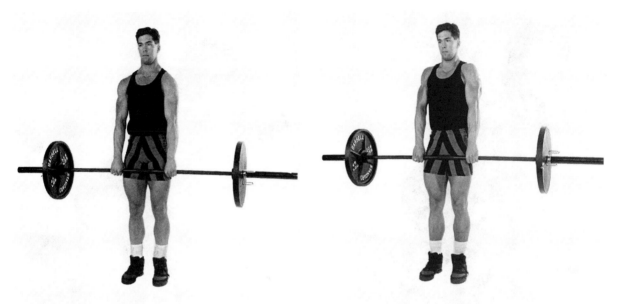

CORRECT TECHNIQUE

Starting Position   Stand erect, your arms straight and hands shoulder-width apart, holding the barbell with an overhand grip.

1. Standing erect throughout the movement, raise your shoulders as high as possible while keeping the arms straight.

2. Lower your shoulders to the starting position. That's a rep.

Standing Dumbbell Press

FOCUS: OUTER AND FRONT DELTOIDS

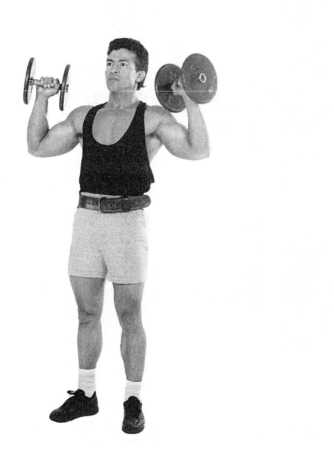 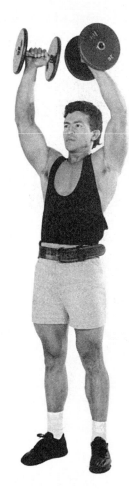

CORRECT TECHNIQUE

Starting Position With your feet shoulder-width apart, stand erect, flexing your abdominals to stabilize the torso. Dumbbells either rest on your shoulders or are supported slightly off your shoulders.

1. Simultaneously press the dumbbells to arm's length. Pause at the top.

2. Simultaneously lower the dumbbells to your shoulders. Repeat the movement the required number of reps.

Standing Lateral Raise

FOCUS: OUTER AND FRONT DELTOIDS

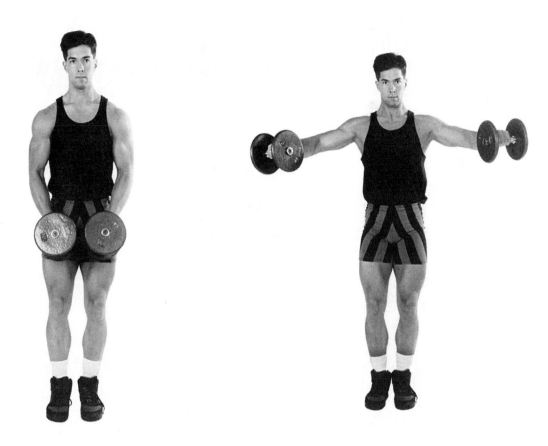

CORRECT TECHNIQUE

Starting Position Stand with your feet shoulder-width apart, dumbbells hanging at your sides with palms facing the thighs. Knees can be slightly bent to maintain balance throughout the movement.

1. Raise the dumbbells through a lateral arc to shoulder height. Keep your arms rigid throughout the movement. The backs of your hands should face the ceiling when dumbbells reach shoulder height.

2. Lower the dumbbells by returning through the same lateral arc to the starting position. That's a rep.

• Elbows may be kept slightly bent, but rigid, throughout the movement. A straight or bent elbow depends on personal taste.

VARIATION: SEATED LATERAL RAISE

MASTER EXERCISE: STANDING LATERAL RAISE

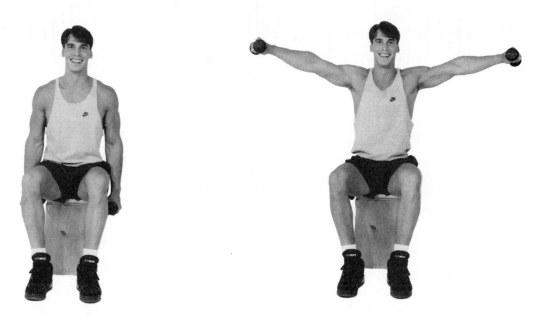

TECHNIQUE VARIATION

- Sit at the end of the bench, back straight, and feet firmly placed on the floor.

Standing Alternate Dumbbell Press

FOCUS: DELTOIDS

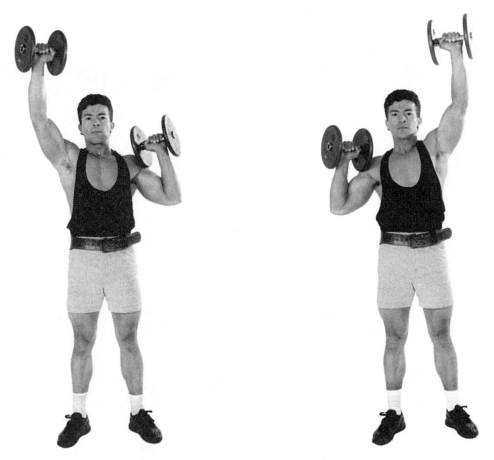

CORRECT TECHNIQUE

Starting Position With feet shoulder-width apart, stand erect, flexing your abdominals to stabilize your torso. Dumbbells should either rest on your shoulders or be supported slightly off your shoulders.

1. Press a dumbbell to arm's length above the head. Pause at the top.

2. Lower the dumbbell while simultaneously pressing the second dumbbell to arm's length above your head. Repeat the movement the required number of reps.

VARIATION: SEATED ALTERNATE DUMBBELL PRESS

MASTER EXERCISE: STANDING ALTERNATE DUMBBELL PRESS

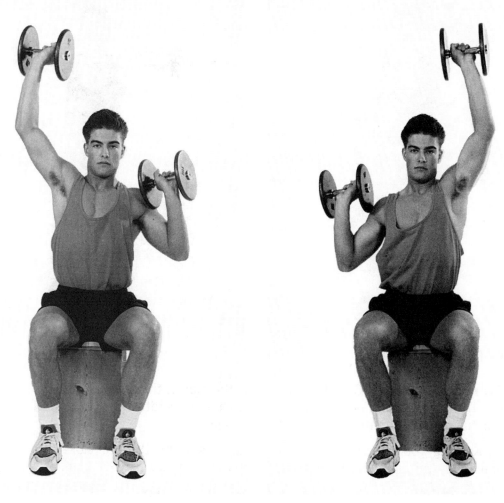

TECHNIQUE VARIATION

• Use the same form as for master exercise, but don't allow the lower back to shift while sitting on the bench. Maintain a straight back and flexed abdominals throughout the exercise movement.

Upright Barbell Row

FOCUS: TRAPEZIUS, DELTOIDS

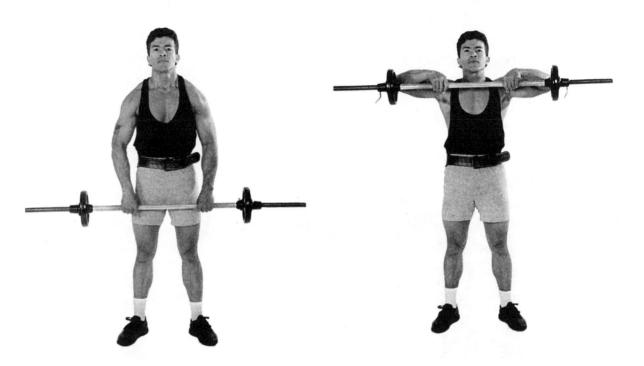

CORRECT TECHNIQUE

Starting Position   Grip the center of the bar with a six-inch-wide overhand grip. Stand erect with your feet shoulder-width apart and the bar hanging from straight arms at your thighs.

1. Keeping your elbows higher than your wrists and the bar close to your body throughout the movement, pull the bar up to your chin.

2. Lower the bar to the starting position. That's a rep.

SPOT TRAINING: THIGHS AND HIPS

Barbell Squat

FOCUS: FRONT OF THIGHS, BUTTOCKS

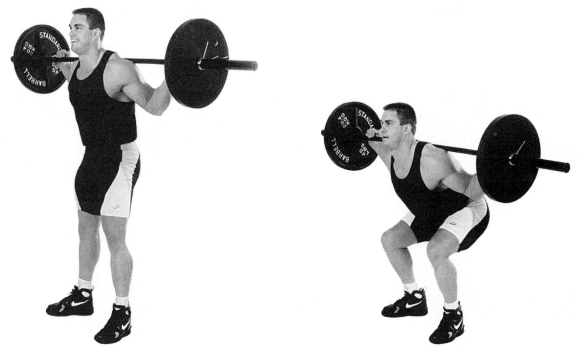

CORRECT TECHNIQUE

Starting Position Stand with your feet shoulder-width apart, bar held in a resting position across your shoulders. Stabilize your torso by isometrically contracting the abdominals and back.

1. Keeping your heels in contact with the floor and eyes forward, lower yourself to the bottom position. Keep your thighs parallel to the floor (or lower) without bending the trunk forward more than necessary (less than 45 degrees).

2. Without pausing at the bottom position, drive up to the starting position. Take care not to bounce or jerk at the bottom position. Although there is technically a stop at the juncture of down and up, the reversal of directions is a smooth transition.

  • Hold your breath throughout the movement, inhaling and exhaling at the top position between repetitions.

VARIATION: FRONT SQUAT
MASTER EXERCISE: BARBELL SQUAT

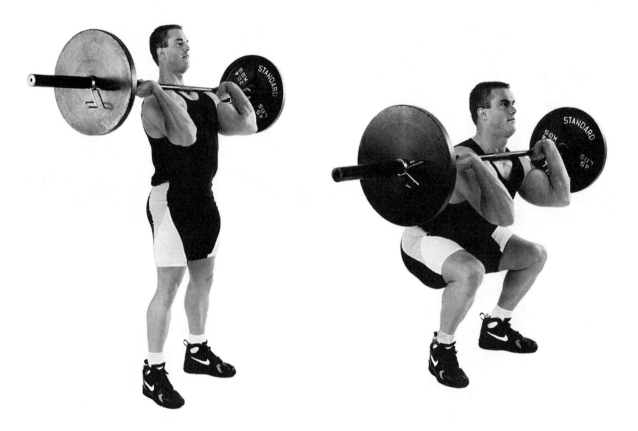

TECHNIQUE VARIATIONS

- Rest the barbell on your upper chest and front deltoids.
- Push your elbows upward and forward to secure the barbell.

VARIATION: FRONT SQUAT TO BENCH

MASTER EXERCISE: BARBELL SQUAT

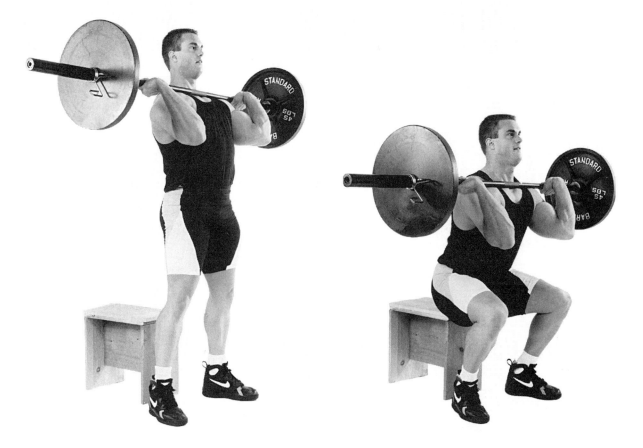

TECHNIQUE VARIATIONS

- Rest the barbell on your upper chest and front deltoids.
- Push your elbows upward and forward to secure the barbell.
- Keeping tension on your thighs, gently touch the bench in the low position before immediately returning to the starting position.

Lunge
FOCUS: FRONT OF THIGHS, HIPS

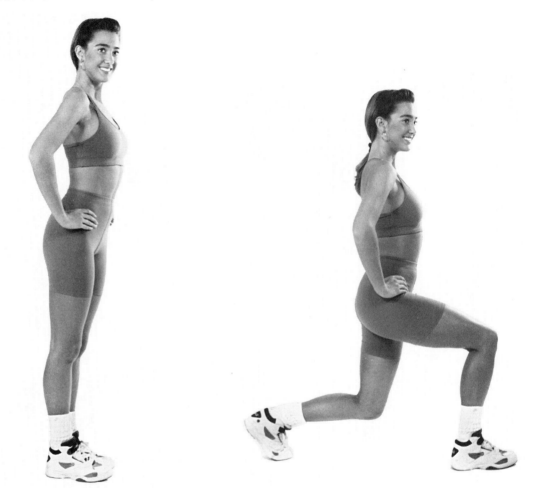

CORRECT TECHNIQUE

Starting Position   Stand upright with feet placed shoulder-width apart.

1. Keeping your head up and back straight, take a long step forward with either foot. Plant your foot and drop your hips until the lead thigh is parallel to the floor. Your knee should be bent approximately 90 degrees and your lead foot should be flat against the floor.

2. Push backward and upward with your lead foot until you are standing erect at the starting position. Repeat with the opposite leg. That's one rep.

VARIATION: LUNGE WITH DUMBBELLS

MASTER EXERCISE: LUNGE

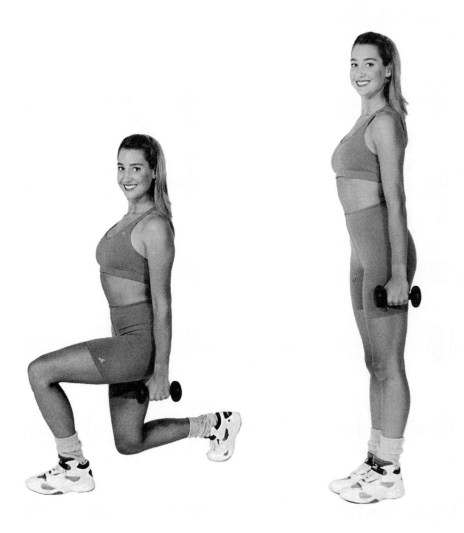

TECHNIQUE VARIATION

• Hold appropriately weighted dumbbells at your sides, palms facing your thighs.

• Once you're able to perfectly execute 10 reps, move up to heavier dumbbells.

Squat Jump

FOCUS: THIGHS

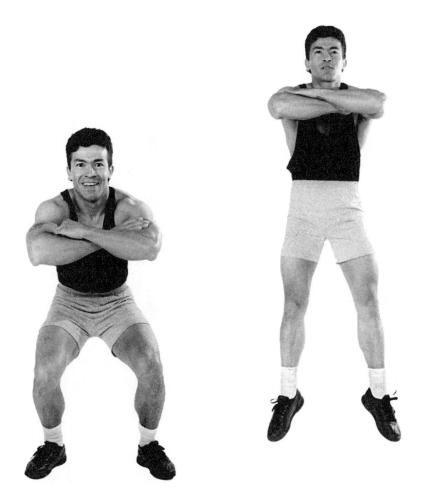

CORRECT TECHNIQUE

Starting Position   Standing erect with your back straight and feet shoulder-width apart, cross your arms over your chest.

1. Squat until your legs are parallel (or lower) with the floor.

2. From a low position, jump into the air as high as possible. Maintain a straight back throughout.

3. Immediately upon landing, control-drop into the starting position. Without pausing, repeat the movement.

Step-ups

FOCUS: FRONT OF THIGHS, HIPS

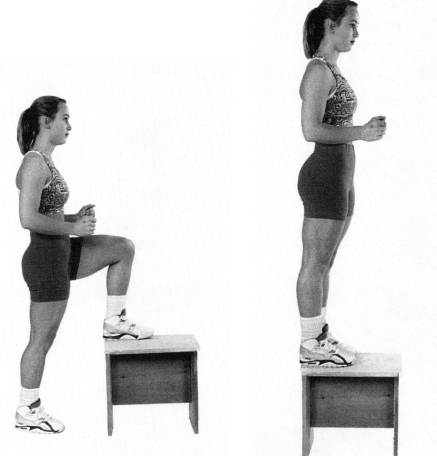

CORRECT TECHNIQUE

Starting Position   Check your bench for stability before beginning this exercise. With feet together, stand facing the *end* of the weight bench.

1. Step up with your right foot, standing erect on top of the bench.

2. Step down to the floor, starting with your left leg and trailing with your right.

3. Repeat the movement, beginning with your left foot this time. Continue to alternate legs until you've completed the required number of reps. That's a set.

VARIATION: STEP-UP WITH DUMBBELLS

MASTER EXERCISE: STEP-UPS

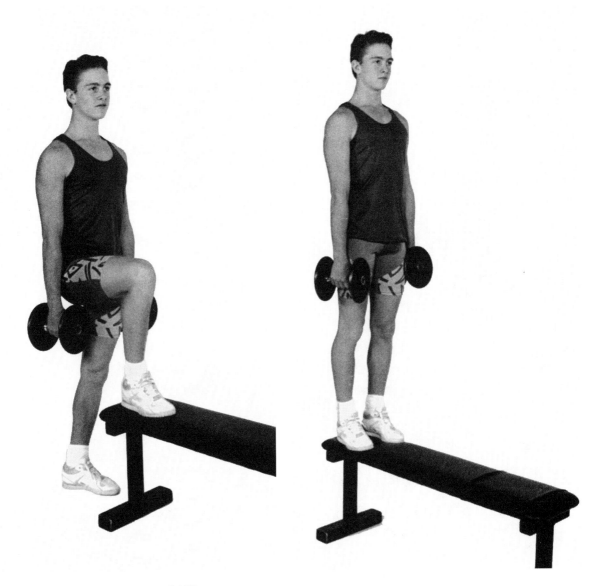

TECHNIQUE VARIATIONS

• Hold appropriate weighted dumbbells at your sides, palms facing your thighs.

• Once you're able to perfectly execute 10 reps, move up to heavier dumbbells.

VARIATION: STEP-UP WITH BARBELL

MASTER EXERCISE: STEP-UPS

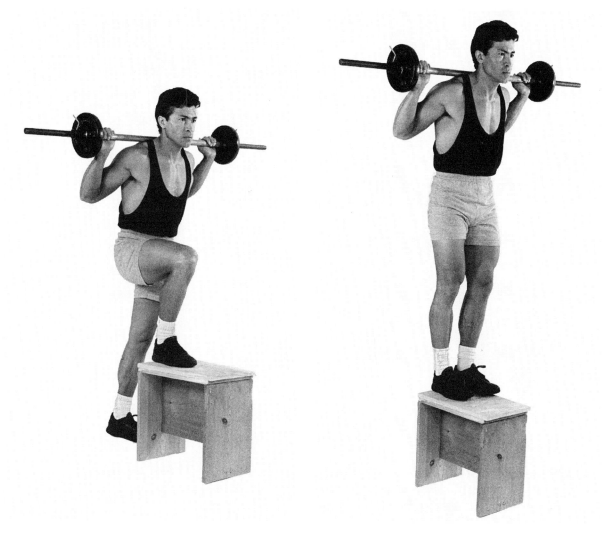

TECHNIQUE VARIATIONS

• Hold an appropriately weighted barbell on your shoulders as pictured, firmly gripping the bar.

• Once you're able to perfectly execute 10 reps, move up to a heavier barbell.

• *Caution:* Barbell step-ups require greater balance than do weightless or dumbbell step-ups. Don't try them until you've mastered the weightless movement.

Deadlift

FOCUS: THIGHS AND BUTTOCKS

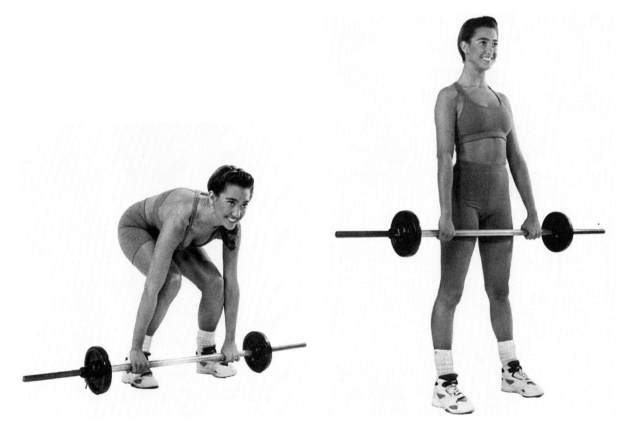

CORRECT TECHNIQUE

Starting Position   Stand with your thighs parallel to the floor, grasping the bar with an overhand grip several inches wider than your shoulder width. Feet are parallel and shoulder-width apart,

1. Keeping your back straight and head up, use your hips, thighs, and lower back to drive upward to a standing position. Pause at the top.

2. Return to the starting position by reversing the motion. That's a rep.

  • Perform the exercise slowly to protect your lower back and take special care not to bounce or jerk the weight at the bottom during the exercise. Emphasize leg action by keeping your back straight and head up. However, be careful not to overemphasize the lower back by straightening your legs more than is absolutely necessary on the rise and return.

Leg Curl
FOCUS: REAR THIGH

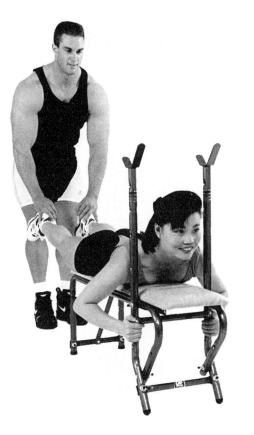 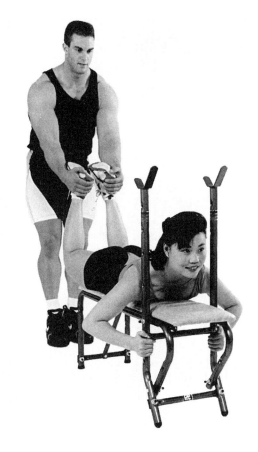

CORRECT TECHNIQUE

Starting Position   Lie facedown on the bench, with your knees at the end of the pad.

1. Without jerking or raising your hips from the bench, bend your legs at the knees, concentrating on the contraction of your hamstrings as your training partner resists your movement.

2. Under control, with your training partner adding resistance, lower to the starting position. That's a rep.

- Many home-gym benches have leg-curl attachments. The technique is the same. The weighted-curl attachment replaces the resistance supplied by a training partner.
- Try one-legged versions of the exercise for variety.

SPOT TRAINING: TRICEPS

Standing Triceps Kick-Back
FOCUS: TRICEPS

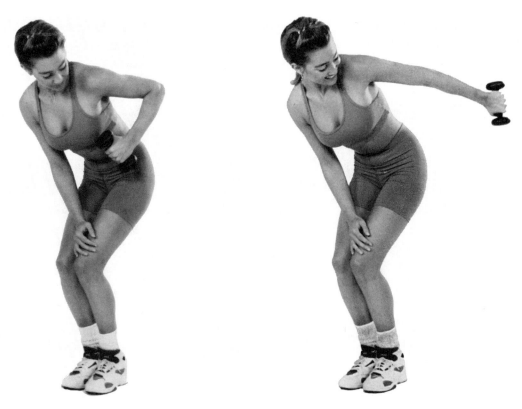

CORRECT TECHNIQUE

Starting Position   Bend forward at the waist with your upper arm held close to your body and parallel with the floor, a dumbbell hanging downward from one hand. Place your free hand on your knee for stability.

1. While keeping your upper arm parallel with the floor, flex your arm until it is straight.

2. Return to the starting position through the same arc, keeping your upper arm parallel to the floor.

• It is important to let your triceps do the work. Don't swing the weight, and always lift under control.

VARIATION: SEATED TRICEP KICK-BACK

MASTER EXERCISE: STANDING TRICEPS KICK-BACK

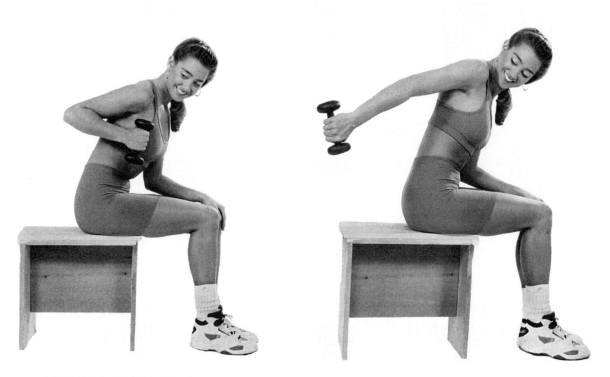

TECHNIQUE VARIATION

- Using the same form as above, sit on the end of a bench bending forward at the waist. Stabilize your torso by placing your hand or forearm on the knee.

Supine Triceps Extension

FOCUS: TRICEPS

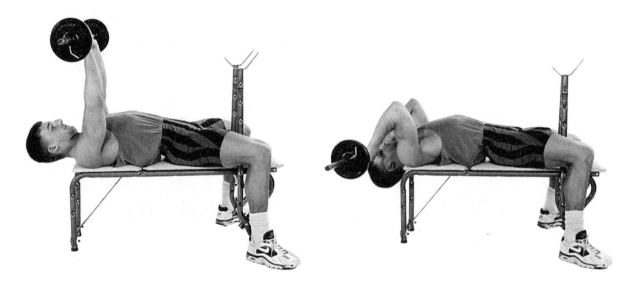

CORRECT TECHNIQUE

Starting Position   Lie on your back either on a bench or on the floor. Grip a barbell with your palms up and your hands spaced six to twelve inches apart. Hold the barbell at arm's length above your shoulders.

1. Keeping your upper arms perpendicular to your torso, lower the bar through an arc until the backs of your hands touch your forehead.

2. Return the barbell through the arc to the starting position, keeping your upper arm perpendicular to your torso throughout the movement. That's a rep.

VARIATION: SUPINE SINGLE-ARM TRICEPS EXTENSION

MASTER EXERCISE: SUPINE TRICEPS EXTENSION

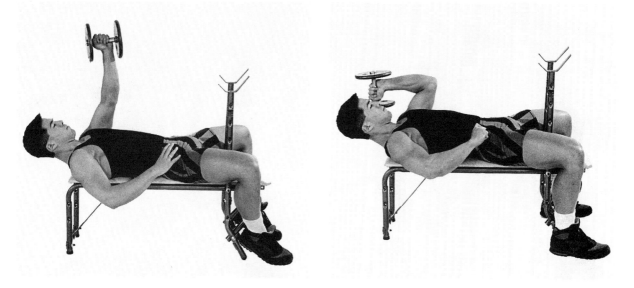

TECHNIQUE VARIATIONS

- Hold a dumbbell in one hand above your shoulder. You may use your free hand to stabilize your working arm if you choose.
- Keeping your upper arm perpendicular with the floor, lower the dumbbell through an arc until it touches your shoulder. Return to the starting position. That's a rep.

Reverse-Grip Bench Press

FOCUS: TRICEPS

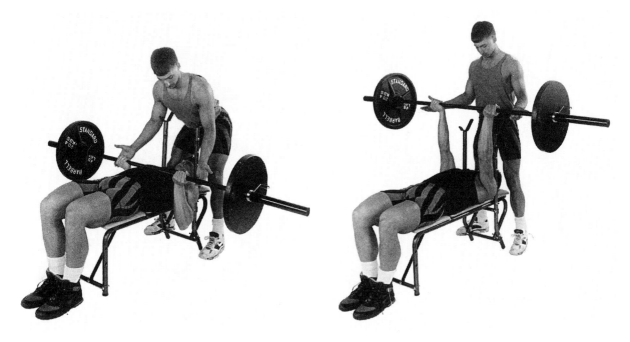

CORRECT TECHNIQUE

Starting Position   Lie on a flat bench with a barbell positioned at arm's length above your shoulders. Hold the barbell securely, palms facing your feet, hands shoulder-width.

1. Lower the bar to your chest, brushing your elbows against the body as the bar descends.

2. Press the barbell to the starting position, keeping your elbows close to the sides of your body as the barbell ascends.

Standing Triceps Press with Barbell

FOCUS: TRICEPS

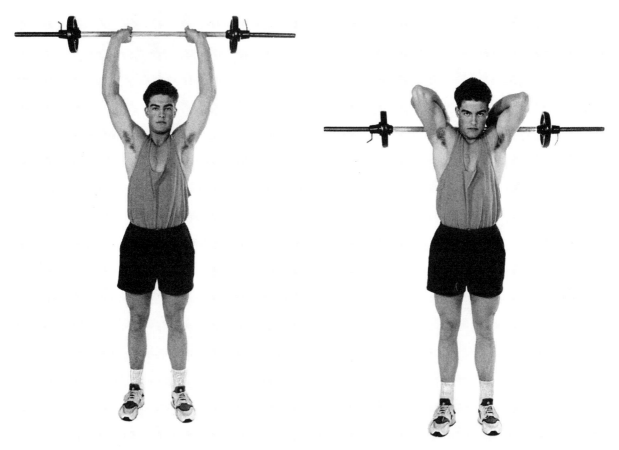

CORRECT TECHNIQUE

Starting Position Hold the bar with a narrow-to-medium-width overhand grip and position the barbell overhead at arm's length.

1. Keeping your upper arms close to your head and perpendicular to the floor, lower the barbell behind your neck in an arc until the motion is restricted by the forearm meeting the biceps.

2. Return to the starting position by flexing the triceps.

• Control the bar throughout the motion. Don't jerk or bounce the bar in the low position or you'll wind up with sore elbows.

VARIATION: STANDING SINGLE-DUMBBELL TRICEPS PRESS

MASTER EXERCISE: STANDING TRICEPS PRESS WITH BARBELL

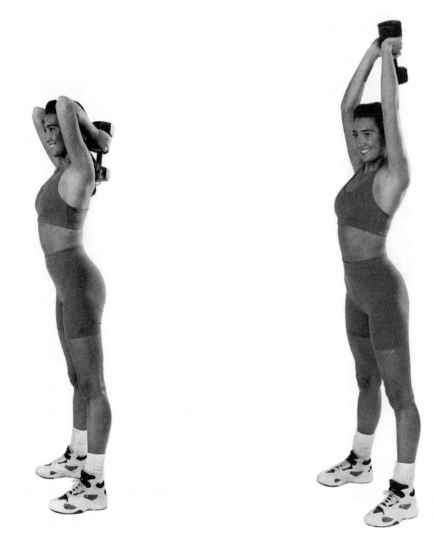

TECHNIQUE VARIATION

• Securely grip a single dumbbell with both hands, holding it arm's length above the head. Follow the remainder of the technique as described in the master exercise.

VARIATION: SEATED SINGLE-DUMBBELL TRICEPS PRESS

MASTER EXERCISE: STANDING TRICEPS PRESS WITH BARBELL

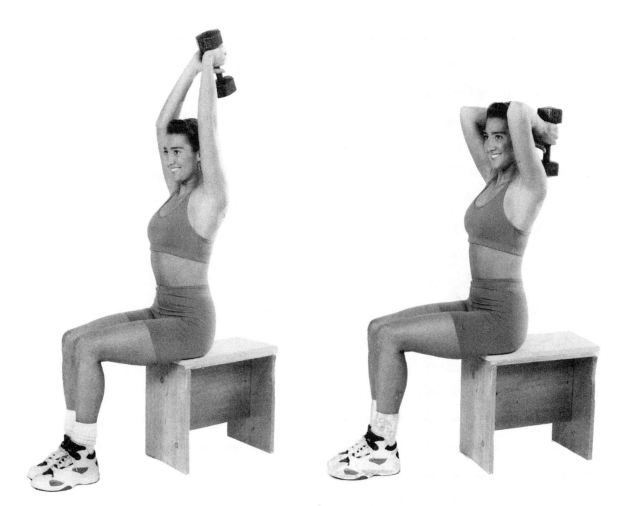

TECHNIQUE VARIATIONS

• Sit on the end of a bench with your feet positioned firmly on the floor.

• Securely grip a single dumbbell with both hands, holding it arm's length above the head. Follow the remainder of the technique as described in the master exercise.

VARIATION: STANDING ONE-ARM TRICEPS PRESS

MASTER EXERCISE: STANDING TRICEPS PRESS WITH BARBELL

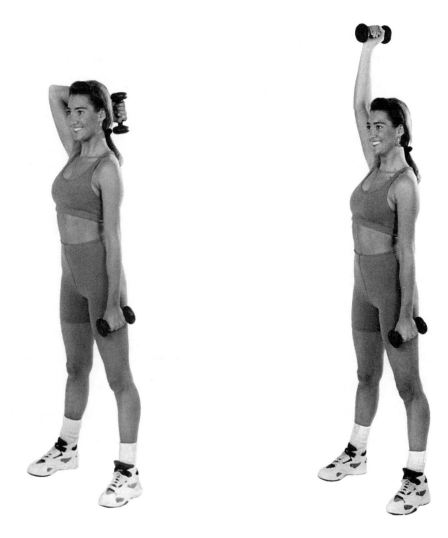

TECHNIQUE VARIATION

• Grip an appropriately weighted dumbbell, holding it with one hand, arm's length above the head. Follow the remainder of the technique as described in the master exercise.

Close-Grip Bench Press

FOCUS: TRICEPS

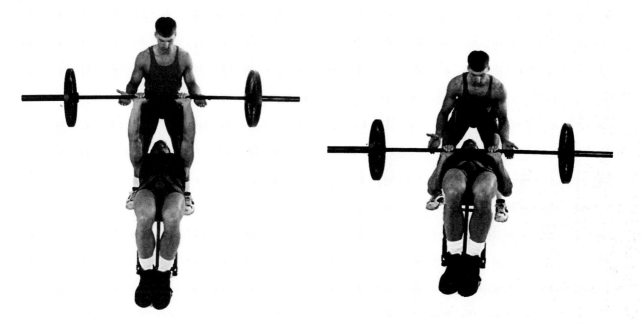

CORRECT TECHNIQUE

Starting Position With your back on the bench, plant your feet firmly on the floor. Support the bar at arm's length with a shoulder-width or narrower grip. Have a knowledgeable spotter in attendance.

1. Your elbows brush your torso as the bar is lowered to your chest.

2. Return to the starting position by pressing the bar upward, fully extending your arms.

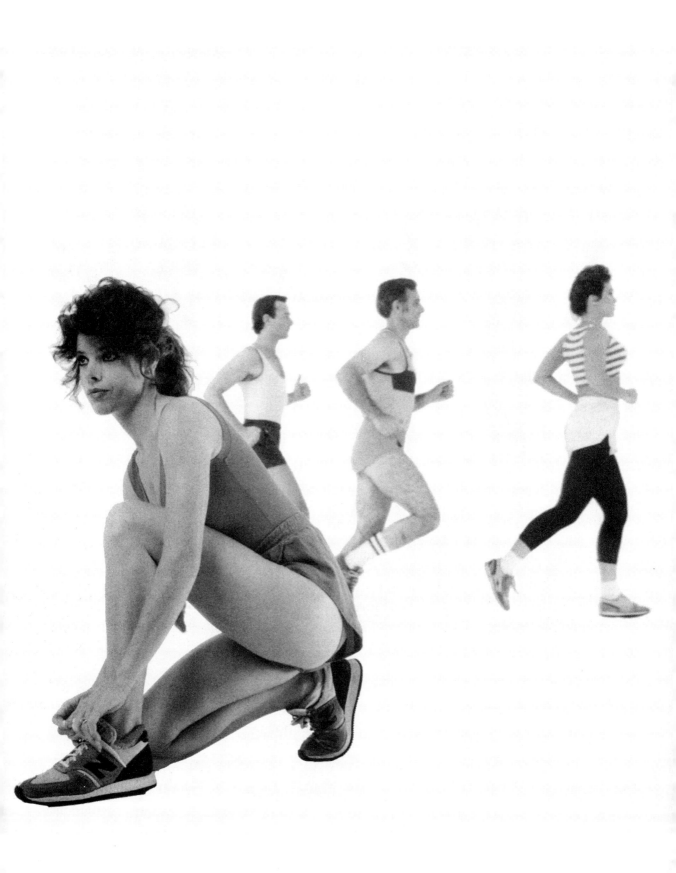

10
SPORTS STRENGTH-TRAINING PROGRAMS

Let's make an imaginary journey to Wimbledon. We're watching Monica Seles as she hits a smashing overhead shot past her opponent.

Years of on-court practice went into perfecting Monica's championship arsenal of shots. But an important off-court training protocol contributed to Monica's success too: Monica weight trained. She weight trained to build strength. Why? Each of Monica's shots requires the coordinated strength of hundreds of her strength-trained muscles. Monica exemplifies the axiom that *a stronger athlete is a better athlete.* That's because strength contributes to the force and speed of every movement she makes on the court.

Monica is one of many examples from the world of professional and amateur sports. For baseball players, boxers, and golfers alike, sport-specific movements strengthened through weight training translate to more powerful and faster movements on the playing field or in the arena. That's a competitive edge.

Sport by sport, this chapter suggests exercises that can strengthen your athletic performance by strengthening the movements of the sport. Here's all you have to do:

• Incorporate the suggested exercises into your basic training program. The suggested exercises strengthen the specific muscles requisite to success in your sport.
• Follow the same training principles, set and rep patterns, and safety precautions as you do for the Basic Workout.

You're on your way to becoming a better athlete!

ARCHERY

"When working to build *strength and tone,* do not try to develop bulk. Large, bulky muscles, though powerful, may not have the suppleness required to withstand the constant stretching and contracting needed for shot after shot. The bulkily muscled person will also have more trouble with string clearance than will a slimmer person."

—John C. Williams, 1972 Olympic gold medal winner and 1984 U.S. Olympic coach

Archery Exercises/Page No.	Primary Movement
1. One-Arm Dumbbell Row/95	• Strengthens the upper back and biceps for the string pull
2. Lunge/92	• Strengthens the hips, thighs, and lower back for stability during the shot.
3. Standard/Close-Grip Bench Press/179	• Strengthens the triceps and shoulders for bow stability
4. Sit-up/99	• Torso stability
5. Stiff-Legged Deadlift/112	• Torso stability

BASEBALL/SOFTBALL

The general demands of the game require that the entire body be strengthened. But developing specific skills requires specific strength-training exercises.

Your Basic Workout will cover general strength demands. The following exercises, selected for a specific goal, are suggested additions to the Basic Workout.

Goal: Better Batting

Baseball Exercises/Page No.	Primary Movement
1. Barbell Wrist Curl/144	• Forearm-wrist-hand strength
2. Reverse Barbell Wrist Curl/145	• Forearm-wrist-hand strength
3. Reverse Trunk Twist/110	• Rotational strength
4. Close-Grip Bench Press/179	• Shoulder and triceps strength

Goal: Better Throwing

Baseball Exercises/Page No.

Primary Movement

1. Supine Triceps Extensions/172
   - Strengthens elbow extension during the throw

2. Upright Barbell Row/158
   - Shoulder strength
3. Bent-Arm Barbell Pullover/140
   - Ball pull-through
4. Dumbbell Wrist Curl/146
   - Ball control

BASKETBALL

Shaquille O'Neal, 1993 NBA Rookie of the Year, is seven feet tall and weights 300 pounds—and he's strong for his size. Watching him play, it is apparent that strength has played an important role in Shaquille's basketball success.

Watching him post up prior to slamming the ball through the net, or establishing a strong defensive position, it's obvious that it is his strength that separates him from the other players on the court. Put another way, the weaker players just plain can't compete with him.

Improved strength improves fundamental basketball skills. That's as true for a weekend player as it is for Shaquille. Improved strength produces quicker passes, higher jumps, and stronger picks, and increases shooting range and accuracy. In short, improved strength improves every aspect of the game.

Basketball Exercises/Page No.

Primary Movement

1. Barbell Squat/159
   - Strengthens jumping muscles of the lower back and thighs

2. Lunge/92
   - Strengthens jumping muscles of the lower back, calf, and thighs

3. Close-Grip Bench Press/179
   - Upper-body shooting muscles
4. Stiff-Legged Deadlift/112
   - Lower-back jumping muscles
5. Leg Raise/107, 109
   - Knee lift during jumping
6. Donkey Toe Raise/127
   - Strengthens jumping muscles of calf

BOWLING

A bowling ball weighs between nine and sixteen pounds. More than 130 muscles make a coordinated effort in a typical ball delivery. Strengthening those 130 muscles can improve technique and impart greater force on the ball as it speeds down the alley, making for greater pin action.

Bowling Exercises/Page No.	Primary Movement
1. Lunge/92	• Hip and leg thrust for the approach and delivery
2. Pull-up/114	• Shoulder girdle, back, and biceps strength during delivery
3. Sit-up/99	• Torso stabilization during delivery
4. Stiff-Legged Deadlift/112	• Torso stabilization
5. Dumbbell Wrist Curl/146	• Ball control during delivery

BOXING

Evander Holyfield, a natural 175-pound light heavyweight, added thirty-five pounds of muscle through weight training to become heavyweight champion of the world. Unfortunately, he discovered that added muscle does not necessarily equate to increased punching power. To be effective, bulk must be added to the muscles that power the punch.

Bigger biceps don't do anything to power the right cross. The biceps don't power any straight punch. The triceps do that. Hence, building bigger biceps is a waste of training time and energy.

A strong right cross begins with leg drive, followed by hip rotation, and finally an extension of the arm from the shoulder. In short, there are muscles from the toes to the fingers involved in the punch. And there are muscles from toes to fingers that aren't. It's important to build the *right* muscles.

If you're a competitive boxer, or just enjoy hitting a heavy bag, incorporate the following exercises into your strength routine to ensure that you're working the right muscles.

Boxing Exercises/Page No.
1. Squat Jump/164
2. Close-Grip Bench Press/179
3. Front Squat/160
4. Reverse Trunk Twist/110
5. Standing Alternate Dumbbell Press/156

Primary Movement
• Leg and hip drive
• Shoulder and triceps strength
• Leg and hip drive
• Rotational force of torso
• Shoulder and triceps strength

CYCLING

Long-Distance Cycling recommended weight training for all cyclists after reviewing recent studies indicating that cycling potential is directly related to leg strength. Quoting David Martin of the Olympic Training Center, the book says, "If your legs are too weak to drive your heart and lungs to maximum levels, your max VO_2 performance will be low. Strengthen your legs and you can improve your peak VO_2 and your cycling performance."

Strength training is also important in preventing injuries. For example, a stronger shoulder girdle and neck can better withstand overuse injuries and absorb crash trauma. Strengthening the quadriceps and hamstrings helps prevent muscle pulls and tears during sprints and hill climbs.

Cycling involves a combination of aerobic, strength, and muscular endurance. Muscular and aerobic endurance is best achieved through on-road cycling or with a variable-resistance exercycle. Strength is most readily improved through weight training.

Cycling Exercises/Page No.
1. Front Squat/160
2. Deadlift/168
3. Step-up/165
4. Reverse Trunk Twist/110
5. Stiff-Legged Deadlift/112

Primary Movement
• Leg drive
• Overall strength
• Leg drive
• Torso power and stabilization
• Lower-back strength/injury prevention

FENCING

The lunge is the most important offensive movement in fencing. That movement can be precisely mimicked during a weight-training movement also called the lunge. Improved strength during the weight-training movement translates to improved strength during the sporting movement as a faster, more powerful lunge.

Fencing Exercises/Page No.	Primary Movement
1. Lunge/92	• Speed, force, and stability of the lunge.
2. Close-Grip Bench Press/179	• Strengthens the shoulders and triceps for a foil thrust
3. Stiff-Legged Deadlift/112	• Strengthens back for torso stabilization
4. Barbell Wrist Curl/144	• Strengthens forearm for foil control
5. Reverse Barbell Wrist Curl/145	• Strengthens forearm for foil control

FOOTBALL

Football was the first team sport to unequivocally endorse weight training as an important training tool. Football players and strength training go hand in hand. The average Division I college football player has lifted weights for six years before he enters college.

Football demands that the force of the legs travel through the torso and continue through the shoulder girdle and arms. That means a need for full-body strength. The following workout recommendations reflect this, and it's really the Basic Workout all over again—with a little more for the legs and back.

Football Exercises/Page No.	Primary Movement
1. Barbell Squat/159	• Hip and leg drive
2. Step-up/165	• Hip and leg drive
3. Deadlift/168	• Back; hip and leg drive
4. Standing Barbell Press/148	• Shoulder girdle thrust
5. Stiff-Legged Deadlift/112	• Back extension
6. Reverse Trunk Twist/110	• Torso stability and rotation
7. Sit-up/99	• Torso stability and power transfer from the hips to the shoulder girdle

GOLF

Every duffer knows that a golf swing demands timing, a virtual symphony of muscular movements. From the backswing to the follow-through, the majority of your 600-plus muscles at some point contribute to the power and timing of an effective swing. Strengthening all those muscles requires a full-body strength-training program. Nick Faldo advises amateur players to "strengthen your leg action. The legs are among the most neglected areas of the swing. Whenever I get the opportunity to watch amateurs play golf, I'm always struck by the instability of their leg action." In short, a modified Basic Workout that emphasizes leg power and torso rotation is the program for you. Include the following exercises if they aren't already part of your regular routine.

Golf Exercises/Page No.	Primary Movement
1. Lunge/92	• Leg and hip drive
2. Step-up/165	• Leg and hip drive
3. Reverse Trunk Twist/110	• Torso rotation during swing
4. Stiff-Legged Deadlift/112	• Torso stabilization during swing
5. Barbell Wrist Curl/144	• Club action (forearm strength)
6. Reverse Barbell Wrist Curl/145	• Club action (forearm strength)
7. Close-Grip Bench Press/179	• Triceps and shoulder action

MARTIAL ARTS

Martial arts—I know it sounds like a broken record—demands a full-body workout to strengthen all the skeletal muscles. But special consideration must be given to the rotation-dependent and kicking movements specific to martial-arts training and competition. With that noted, be sure to make the following exercises part of your training routine.

Martial Arts Exercises/Page No.	Primary Movement
1. Reverse Trunk Twist/110	• Torso and hip rotation
2. Leg Raise/107, 109	• Knee lift during kick; torso stabilization
3. Close-Grip Bench Press/179	• Punching action

RACQUET SPORTS

"Don't just accept the ravages of age. Keep your body in shape with weight training."

—Jim Loehr, *Tennis* magazine, January 1993

Jim Loehr's advice for older tennis players applies to any athlete wanting to keep a competitive edge. It applies to racquetball and squash players, too.

All three racquet sports share similar movements and strength demands.

Let's imagine the swing as an example. The force of the swing begins with leg drive, moves through the rotation of the hips and torso, and is finally delivered to the ball through the muscles of the shoulder girdle, arm, and hand. Muscles from toe to fingertip add to the swing.

That's why the racquet sports require a full-body program—the Basic Workout. Ivan Lendl and many other players use weight training to increase power and to prevent injuries. Certain biomechanical factors specific to racquet sports demand that the exercises listed below be included in that program.

Racquet Sport Exercises/Page No.	Primary Movement
1. Lunge/92	• Lunge at ball
2. Step-up/165	• Leg and hip drive
3. Reverse Trunk Twist/110	• Rotation of the torso and hips
4. Barbell Wrist Curl/144	• Wrist action and grip
5. Reverse Barbell Wrist Curl/145	• Wrist action
6. Bent-Arm Barbell Pullover/140	• Overhand swing

RUNNING AND JOGGING

In the book *Run Fast,* Dr. David Costill, director of the Human Performance Laboratory at Ball State University, says, "Use your weights mainly for a supplemental maintenance program. Go through a routine that stresses most of your muscles. Once in a while, push yourself. That should be enough strength and endurance for most runners."

Distance running is less affected by strength training than perhaps any other recreational or competitive sport. That's most obvious when considering the physiques of champion marathoners. Running depends much more heavily on aerobic capacity than on muscular strength.

But strength training does have an important place in the distance runner's training scheme by reducing the risk of injury. A stronger ankle is less likely sprained when stepping on a rock. A stronger knee is less likely damaged when running off a curb.

Strength training can also prevent the emaciating muscle loss of a runner whose body must scavenge noninvolved tissue to satisfy the energy demands of too much running.

What strength-training workout is best for the distance runner and jogger? The Basic Workout, because it works the whole body, preventing any wholesale muscle loss from the energy demands of the track or highway.

Invest twenty to forty minutes, three days per week, and you'll keep your shoulders, arms, chest, and the shape of your derriere while running as much as you like. Stick with the Basic Workout.

SKIING

Ask any seasonal skier. Skiing requires the stamina of a distance runner and the strength of a football player. Hence, getting ready for the ski season means an off-season strength program and an aerobic conditioning program.

A step-aerobics class combined with a weight-training program will prepare you for the slopes or the woods.

Make the following strength-training exercises part of your workout routine.

Skiing Exercises/Page No.	Primary Movement
1. Front Squat/160	• Leg and hip drive
2. Close-Grip Bench Press/179	• Pole action
3. Stiff-Legged Deadlift/112	• Stability of lower back and hips
4. Sit-up/99	• Torso stability
5. Lunge/92	• Leg and hip drive
6. Leg Raise/107, 109	• Knee lift
7. Bent-Arm Barbell Pullover/140	• Pole action

SWIMMING

Twenty-year-old swimmer Summer Sanders, winner of four medals at the 1992 Barcelona Olympics, regularly weight-trains to supplement her rigorous swim practices.

Prior to the Olympic Games, Sanders weight-trained six days a week, Monday through Saturday, about an hour a day. This was on top of her daily two-hour swim.

Good swimmers like Sanders are strong. Propulsion through the water is dependent on the strength of the swimmer's muscles. Stronger muscles propel you more quickly through the water.

The value of weight training is universal; sprinters and distance swimmers alike make use of it. Each has more power available for successive strokes, resulting in faster times at every distance.

Swimming strokes differ. No one training routine is perfect for all strokes. But the following exercises will benefit all strokes.

Swimming Exercises/Page No.
1. Pull-up/114
2. Sit-up/99
3. Step-up/165
4. Stiff-Legged Deadlift/112
5. Push-up/128

Primary Movement
- Upper-body pulling motions
- Torso stabilization
- General leg-movement strength
- Injury prevention to lower back
- Upper-body thrust

VOLLEYBALL

Volleyball players must jump and spike throughout a game. Superior leg strength as well as strong abdominal and back muscles contribute to successful play. Consistent weight training will also prevent muscle tears and strains in this sport where the players are constantly contracting the back and leg muscles.

Volleyball Exercises/Page No.
1. Pull-up/114
2. Sit-up/99
3. Step-up/165
4. Standing Single-Leg Toe Raise/125
5. Lunge/92

Primary Movement
- Upper-body pulling motions
- Torso stabilization
- General leg-movement strength
- Jumping

- Jumping and lunging

APPENDIX

DATE																					
EXERCISE	r	w	r	w	r	w	r	w	r	w	r	w	r	w	r	w	r	w	r	w	r

NAME

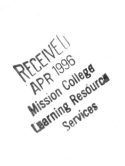